HEALING TO ALL THEIR FLESH

ALSO BY JEFF LEVIN

Divine Love: Perspectives from the World's Religious Traditions
(Edited with Stephen G. Post)

Faith, Medicine, and Science: A Festschrift in Honor of Dr. David B. Larson
(Edited with Harold G. Koenig)

Religion in the Lives of African Americans: Social, Psychological, and Health Perspectives
(with Robert Joseph Taylor and Linda M. Chatters)

God, Faith, and Health: Exploring the Spirituality-Healing Connection

Essentials of Complementary and Alternative Medicine
(Edited with Wayne B. Jonas)

Religion in Aging and Health: Theoretical Foundations and Methodological Frontiers
(Edited)

ALSO BY KEITH G. MEADOR

Heal Thyself: Spirituality, Medicine, and the Distortion of Christianity (with Joel James Shuman)

Growing Old in Christ
(Edited with Stanley Hauerwas, Carole Bailey Stoneking, and David Cloutier)

HEALING TO ALL THEIR FLESH

Jewish and Christian Perspectives on Spirituality, Theology, and Health

JEFF LEVIN, PHD
KEITH G. MEADOR, MD

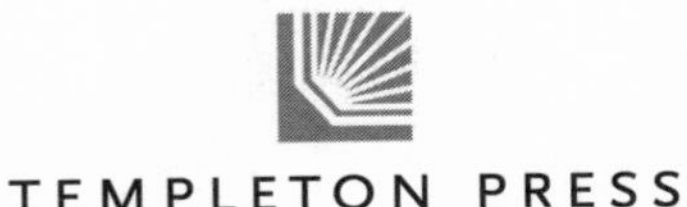

TEMPLETON PRESS

Templeton Press
300 Conshohocken State Road, Suite 500
West Conshohocken, PA 19428
www.templetonpress.org

Designed and typeset by Kachergis Book Design

Library of Congress Cataloging-in-Publication Data
Healing to all their flesh : Jewish and Christian perspectives on spirituality, theology, and health / [edited by] Jeff Levin, Keith G. Meador.
p. cm.
Includes bibliographical references and index.
ISBN 978-1-59947-375-8 (pbk. : alk. paper) — ISBN 978-1-59947-419-9 (e-book)
1. Health—Religious aspects—Christianity. 2. Health—Religious aspects—Judaism. 3. Healing—Religious aspects—Christianity. 4. Healing—Religious aspects—Judaism. 5. Aging—Religious aspects—Christianity. 6. Aging—Religious aspects—Judaism. I. Levin, Jeffrey S. II. Meador, Keith G.
BT732.H39 2012
201´.661—dc23
2012010234

Printed in the United States of America

12 13 14 15 16 17 10 9 8 7 6 5 4 3 2 1

For Lea, great and wise healer (J. L.)

For Patricia in memory, and
Katie in hope (K. G. M.)

CONTENTS

Foreword ix
Rabbi Samuel E. Karff, DHL

Acknowledgments xiii

Prologue. The Intersection of Spirituality, Theology, and Health 3
Jeff Levin

PART 1: JEWISH PERSPECTIVES

1. Cure and Healing, Where God Met Science: Four Decades of Spiritual Progress 17
William Cutter

2. Contemplating a Theology of Healthy Aging 26
Richard Address

3. Dwindling or Grateful: Toward a Resilient Old Age 52
Dayle A. Friedman

4. Using Jewish Law to Respond to Contemporary Issues in Bioethics 65
Elliot N. Dorff

5. Give Me Your Hand: Exploring Judaism's Approach to the Relationship of Spirit and Health 97
Simkha Y. Weintraub

PART 2: CHRISTIAN PERSPECTIVES

6. St. Thomas Aquinas and the End(s) of Religion, Spirituality, and Health 123
Warren Kinghorn

7. Beguiling Religion: The Bifurcations and Biopolitics of Spirituality and Medicine 150
M. Therese Lysaught

8. The Ontological Generality in Spirituality and Health 186
Stephen G. Post

9. From Health to *Shalom*: Why the Religion and Health Debate Needs Jesus 219
John Swinton

10. *Suffering Presence*: Twenty-Five Years Later 242
Stanley Hauerwas

Epilogue. Theology and Health: Challenges and Possibilities 259
Keith G. Meador

About the Contributors 271

Index 273

FOREWORD

To fully appreciate this important volume, a historical perspective may be helpful. Before physicians constituted a distinct profession, the roles of physical and spiritual healer were imbedded in the biblical priest or shaman. Even after there were physicians, Hippocrates taught that if the patient liked and trusted the doctor and believed in the efficacy of his healing acts, treatment was likely to be more effective. The early synagogue and church believed that God, the ultimate healer, endowed the physician with his healing power. By the middle of the twentieth century, new diagnostic tools, pharmaceutical "magic bullets," and advances in surgery gave rise to a biomedical paradigm of medical education and practice. The physician's relation to God or to the patient was no longer considered intrinsically relevant to the healing process. The knowledge and skills associated with the new biomedicine was solely determinative of medical outcome.

Some thirty years later, the vaunted biomedical model was deemed inadequate. Patients complained of having too much contact with the cold steel of diagnostic tests in relation to the time they were able to tell their story and be listened to by their doctor. A significant number yearned for a competent biomedical clinician who was also a healer.

At this time, science provided us with a more sophisticated appreciation of the mind-body connection. (Medical researchers were now able to track the effect of uncontrolled stress in weakening the immune system.) This helped spawn a biopsychosocialspiritual model of medical education and practice. Over the next decade or so, more than one hundred medical centers in the United States created programs in "holistic medicine," "medical humanities," or "spirituality and medicine."

During this period many research studies found a positive correlation between a patient's involvement in a religious community, including regular public worship, and faster recovery from surgery, better coping with chronic illness and mental illness, and even a longer life span. Of course these findings did not establish an ontological claim for the reality of a God who answers prayer. The Holy One does not submit to an experimental design. Rather, such studies confirm the reality of the mind-body connection: how our mind frames the world can affect, for better or worse, what happens in our bodies.

Generally, this research was done and analyzed by social scientists, not theologians. The importance of this volume derives from the thoughtful, theologically informed observations its editors solicited from Jewish and Christian respondents.

Certain commonalities between the two groups of contributors will readily become apparent. Caring for our bodies is a religious obligation, but physical fitness as an all-consuming end in itself is too limited to validate a human life. Good health becomes spiritually resonant when it leads us to love and glorify God and (Jewish idiom) to partner with our Creator to heal brokenness in that tiny corner of God's world entrusted to our care. The spiritually attuned physician will acknowledge that his or her power to heal is finite. Since no amount of medical technology will enable us to shed our mortality, the physician must discern and respect the boundary between extending life and prolonging dying.

The attentive reader will perceive some difference between the Jewish and Christian attitude toward suffering. Warren Kinghorn writes that "the body the church presents to be cared for is . . . shaped by practices carried by the story of God in which . . . even our suffering can be a gift that makes more intimate our relation with God and one another." In Judaism, suffering is less a redemptive gift to be cherished than the price of living as an embodied creature and, too often, the price of serving God in a world not yet redeemed. Wherever possible, suffering is something to be relieved.

Both Jewish and Christian contributors favor a spirituality deeply rooted in the particular beliefs, narratives, and disciplines of the great historic traditions over a free floating generic spirituality. They also validate a religion and health program which defines a human flourishing and wholeness that also embraces those who will not be physically cured in this world.

This volume will amply reward its readers. The editors deserve our praise and gratitude for adding a rich and significant dimension to the religion and health literature.

Rabbi Samuel E. Karff, DHL
Houston, Texas

ACKNOWLEDGMENTS

The editors would like to express their deepest gratitude to the ten chapter authors of the insightful and heartfelt essays contributed to *Healing to All Their Flesh*. It was great joy to read each of these chapters as they arrived; we experienced a growing sense of excitement as we began to recognize the remarkable caliber of scholarly works that we had been blessed to receive. This book project was somewhat of an experiment: what would happen, we wondered, if we identified leading Jewish rabbinic and Christian theological scholars who have written at the intersection of religion, faith, and spirituality, on the one hand, and health, healing, medicine, and health care, on the other, then brought them together and gave them carte blanche to say whatever they had ever wished to say on the subject, from any angle? The results far exceeded our expectations.

We have long believed that the continued emergence of a research field at the intersection of religion and health has been worse off for not having elicited the input of theological, pastoral, bioethical, and religious scholars and academic clergy. Existing studies, on the whole, read as if constructed in a vacuum, devoid of any theoretical or conceptual contexts that actually reflect the religious life of real people. This is not to call into question the motives or expertise of the clinicians, social and behavioral scientists, and epidemiologists who have conducted most of this research. The two of us, between us, wear all of these hats and have conducted some of this research. We and our cherished colleagues are, for the most part, doing the best we can with what has mostly been research projects based on existing data and existing measures typically collected for other purposes. But, still, to wonder about and to investigate in earnest what is, essentially, the relation of spirit and flesh—a question of profundity that has challenged the greatest minds for thousands of years—and to do so without consulting the perspectives of those scholars whose bailiwick is the human spirit seems, well, odd or misguided, at best, and perhaps downright foolish, at worst.

This project has focused on the two faith traditions that we know best: Judaism and Christianity. The contributors represent, amongst them, much of the breadth of these two traditions, denominationally, but of course given the brevity of this volume not every Christian communion or Jewish movement is covered. We are content, though, because these chapters were not written as explicit denominational statements, but rather as personal statements reflecting varied and long-standing interests among these esteemed authors. Perhaps down the road, we will follow up this project with a companion volume containing the perspectives of representative theological scholars from a larger sweep of the world's religious traditions.

We would also like to extend our thanks to the wonderful folks at Templeton Press who helped to make this book project such a success. Natalie Lyons Silver, our terrific editor, is talented, helpful, and patient. The lead editor, Jeff Levin, worked with Natalie on a prior book, *Divine Love*, and in the acknowledgments of that book noted that Natalie "has been a delight to work with and is an author's dream: friendly, knowledgeable, hardworking, detail-oriented, understanding, accessible." Three years later, this description still holds and his esteem for her has only grown. Thank you, Natalie. Thanks, too, goes out to Susan Arellano, Templeton Press publisher, for believing in this book, and to the many others at Templeton Press who have helped us throughout the writing, editing, publishing, and marketing phases of this project.

In addition, we would like to thank our work colleagues for their support during the editing of this book. For Jeff Levin, this includes Byron Johnson and Rod Stark, codirectors of the Institute for Studies of Religion at Baylor University, and Elizabeth Davis, Baylor provost, who have graciously provided him with a welcoming academic home that has enabled him to pursue scholarly projects that are well outside the mainstream of his profession, epidemiology. He also wishes to thank the fantastic administrative staff at the Institute: Frances Malone, Cameron Andrews, and Leone Moore. For Keith Meador, this includes colleagues in the Center for Biomedical Ethics and Society and the Department of Psychiatry at Vanderbilt University and the sustaining conversations on these issues with friends over the last twenty years.

Finally, Jeff also wishes to acknowledge Michele Prince and Adi Bodenstein, treasured colleagues at the Kalsman Institute on Judaism and Health located at Hebrew Union College-Jewish Institute of Religion. The three of us have partnered on several projects, including the Kalsman Roundtable on Judaism and Health Research, which facilitated Jeff's work on the present book.

To close, we would like to thank our families for their love and support. Jeff would like to thank his beloved wife, best friend, and fellow epidemiologist, Lea Steele Levin. Keith thanks his children, Hannah, John, and Catherine, along with Katie, who brings hope and delight into his life daily. We pray that *Healing to All Their Flesh* will encourage a new commitment to dialogue among scientists, clinicians, and theological scholars to the benefit, ultimately, of all of us.

HEALING TO ALL THEIR FLESH

JEFF LEVIN

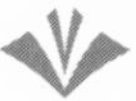

PROLOGUE. THE INTERSECTION OF SPIRITUALITY, THEOLOGY, AND HEALTH

> My son, be attentive to my words; incline your ear to my sayings. Let them not escape from your sight; keep them within your heart. For they are life to those who find them, and healing to all their flesh.[1]

The past quarter century has seen a flowering of scientific research on the intersection of religion and health.[2] While scholarly writing and one-off studies on this subject actually date to the nineteenth century,[3] only in the past couple of decades have empirical research and writing grown to become a recognized niche within academic science and medicine. This field—and there is growing reason to consider this area a field—is quickly losing its earlier identity as a marginal topic and is becoming institutionalized into the mainstream of several disciplines and specialties. These include medical sociology, health psychology, social gerontology, psychosocial epidemiology, and the medical specialties of geriatrics, family medicine, and psychiatry. An early literature review of published research on religion and health, as of the mid-1980s, found about 200 studies. The first edition of the *Handbook of Religion and Health*, published in 2001, found 1,200 studies along with another 400 scholarly papers.[4] The forthcoming second edition of the *Handbook* will identify somewhere north of 3,000 published studies and untold additional thousands of scholarly essays, reviews, reports, and commentaries.[5] To call the growth of scientific research on this subject exponential would not be hyperbole.

As summarized in numerous review essays, systematic reviews, and meta-analyses, the scope of published empirical findings is broad and deep. Large programs of epidemiologic, social, behavioral, and clinical research have identified salutary effects of religious identity and practice in relation to numerous personal and population health indicators of both physical and mental health. These include especially large, systematic bodies of significant findings linking dimensions of religiousness to lower rates of morbidity and mortality due to heart disease, hypertension, cerebrovascular disease, and overall and site-specific cancer, and to a lower incidence of psychiatric disorders such as depression, anxiety, suicide, psychosis, and substance abuse. Numerous studies also point to a strong protective effect with respect to physical disability and overall longevity, and implicate religion as an important factor for general well-being and quality of life, according to various measures. Moreover, these findings have emerged, consistently, for many decades regardless of the age, gender, race or ethnicity, socioeconomic status, nationality, or religious affiliation of respondents, or the study design employed, or how religiousness is conceived of and assessed.

Clearly, these studies, and this field, did not emerge from a vacuum. But from the way that many contemporary research studies on religious factors in health are designed—the questions addressed (reasonable or not), the conceptual approaches to assessing religiousness (sensible or not), the literature cited (or uncited), the theoretical frameworks and hypotheses (or lack thereof) underlying analyses—this point is not obvious. It is increasingly evident to those of us who were around when this field began to emerge twenty-five years ago that much of the scholarly writing being done today, and indeed most of the empirical research, is coming from investigators who are newly discovering this subject and who are moving forward with their own studies without a significant context for this work. That is, a putative relationship between religious involvement and personal or population health is being treated especially by sociomedical and biomedical researchers as simply another garden-variety topic for sophisticated analysis. Religion is just more grist for the mill of structural-equation models, survival analyses, logistic regressions, and the like. So much effort is focused on the narrow details of respective studies and the application of cutting-edge methodologies and hardly any on the sorts of metaphilosophical questions (e.g., "What does this really mean?") that occupied early investigators.

The novelty and marginality of studying religion in a health or medical context actually worked to the advantage of those pioneers back in the day who were seeking to construct a field: it led them to be deliberate and focus (if somewhat) on conceptual and theoretical issues and to try to trace the extensive history of the interface of religion and medicine. Today, this novelty and marginality are gone—not a bad thing, by any means—but so, too, it seems is an understanding of the larger context from which religion and health studies evolved.

What is this context?

One, the possibility of a religion-health connection is not a recently hatched idea, despite the insistence of so many researchers and commentators. It has been around for a very long time. Scholarly and scientific writing on this subject has been ongoing for over one hundred years, including well-known commentaries by seminal figures in biomedicine such as Drs. William Osler[6] and John Shaw Billings.[7] Published works in the Christian psychology and pastoral counseling vein date back even further, to the early decades of the nineteenth century. For example, *Observations on the Influence of Religion upon the Health and Physical Welfare of Mankind*,[8] written by Dr. Amariah Brigham, a founder of the American Psychiatric Association, was published in 1835. But discourse on the intersection of theological and biomedical spheres of knowledge is far older still—to wit, the great systems of healing promulgated by medieval and ancient esoteric schools of philosophy and theosophy, across religious and wisdom traditions. These include the writings of initiates of mystery schools and secret brotherhoods, of Gnostics and kabbalists, of adepts of Western and

Eastern mystical traditions, and of shamans and indigenous healers from myriad cultures throughout the world—writings dating back, in some instances, thousands of years.[9]

Today, a vibrant and flourishing intellectual field is in place. Scholarly publications in mainstream peer-reviewed journals are commonplace. Research funding is no longer scarce, including grants from branches of the U.S. National Institutes of Health. Academic research centers and distinguished chairs now exist, developments that just a few years ago would have seemed preposterous. In a way, what we have described has followed much the same trajectory as any other slowly emerging field—think of, say, behavioral medicine twenty-five years ago.

Nevertheless, in the understandable haste to get about one's business, in a research sense, something important has been lost. The field has matured and entered a state of what Kuhn famously termed "normal science,"[10] defined as a status in which a single paradigm or way of making sense of the reality of a given subject (e.g., religion and health) predominates. For Kuhn, this is a critical signpost that a theory or area of inquiry has coalesced into a field qua field. For the study of religion and health, such a state has emerged over the past decade or so.

The result? The study of religion and health has become an accepted and acceptable pursuit and, thus, apparently, there is less perceived need for the kind of reflection and reappraisal that are required of explorers of uncharted terrains. More and more, investigators are focused on the matter at hand—their respective research studies—rather than concerned about the kind of broader issues—of acceptability, context, and field-building—that used to be bandied about. While methodology has been engaged in ever more sophisticated ways, using better and better data sources and analytic procedures—the "what" of research, one might say—theoretical issues have been largely ignored—the "how" and "why" of research. There seems to be a serious disconnect between the sort of information that is accumulating about religion-health interconnections and more fundamental (and one could say existential) questions about the relation of spirit and body that animated discussions of early pioneers in this discourse decades ago.

In 1957, the Academy of Religion and Mental Health of the Blanton-Peale Institute established a forum for "a free interplay of discussion" on themes at the interface of religion, psychiatry, and medicine. Every year or two, more or less, through the 1960s, with support early on from the Josiah Macy Jr. Foundation, a thematic symposium was held that featured lively and groundbreaking interdisciplinary and inter-religious conversation and debate on the potential "acceptance of religion as a professional ally" by clinicians, researchers, and medical educators. The published proceedings of these meetings were some of the earliest programmatic writing on religion and health as a field of study, and they remain among the best and most enlightening of all the scholarly writing that has ever appeared on the subject. These round-tables featured the contributions of preeminent intellectual figures from myriad secular disciplines, including Drs. Abraham H. Maslow, Otto Klineberg, Gordon W. Allport, Karl Menninger, Margaret Mead, and Talcott Parsons, among many others.

The themes, and associated questions, posed at these symposia were important and fascinating, and engendered discussions that would be wisely revisited by today's religion and health investigators. To wit: "Religion, Science, and Mental Health" (held in 1957),[11] "Religion in the Developing Personality" (1958),[12] "Religion, Culture, and Mental Health" (1959),[13] "The Place of Value Systems in Medical Education" (1960),[14] "Research in Religion and Health" (1961),[15] and "Moral Values in Psychoanalysis" (1963).[16] Over half a century after the first of these gatherings, these conversations remain as vital and timely as ever.

Yet, today, could it truly be said that we have fully addressed these and related issues? Have we even made any headway? The present editors believe that while the answer to the second question is "yes, surely," the answer to the first question is "emphatically no." There is, we believe, a reason for this: the striking absence of serious theological engagement in the identification and construction of topics that feed scholarship in this field. This is not an insignificant point. A field ostensibly devoted to the interface of "God, faith, and health,"[17] to quote from the title of a book by one of the editors (J. L.), or of "spirituality, theology, and health," to reference the name of a major academic center formerly codirected by the other editor (K. G. M.), would, one presumes, be highlighted by or at least prominently feature the informed perspectives of leading theological, pastoral, ethical, and religious scholars and academic clergy. If so, one would be wrong.

Things were not always this way. Before the empirical research enterprise that is the contemporary religion and health field got started in earnest, over twenty years ago, theoretical discussions, especially theological discussions, could be found on occasion throughout this literature. These include seminal works by pioneering bioethicist Dr. Kenneth Vaux (in 1976) outlining the theological foundations of how and why, specifically, "religious beliefs and associated moral habits" influence health-related attitudes and behaviors;[18] and by medical and religious historian and bioethicist Dr. Harold Y. Vanderpool (in 1977) on the ways that the Christian faith, through the example of Jesus, has demonstrated that it "is concerned in a unique and intensive way with the health and well-being of human beings."[19] Another significant contribution along these lines, from the social epidemiologist Dr. Berton H. Kaplan (in 1976): a note on biblical, psychoanalytic, and literary themes elucidating the ostensible role of religious beliefs in coronary artery disease.[20] An especially important (and relatively forgotten) discussion was initiated by no less than Dr. Paul Tillich, in his essays, "The Relation of Religion and Health" (from 1946) and "The Meaning of Health" (from 1961), reprinted together in a monograph published in 1981.[21]

Over the past couple of decades, this tradition of writing seems to have faded out. This corresponds, lamentably, to the time period during which empirical research on religion and health has expanded by at least an order of magnitude. Thankfully, however, there are exceptions. One example is found in the work of theologian and epidemiologist Dr. Peter Van Ness. He has penned important works on the rapprochement of religion and medicine, including a recent essay describing theology and epidemiology "as complementary perspectives" for research by gerontologists and geriatricians.[22]

Notwithstanding the happy exceptions, the most honest appraisal of the past two decades of progress in the religion and health field is this: collectively, we have dropped the ball when it comes to a concerted effort to make sense of and draw meaning from the rapidly accumulating evidence that expressions or functions of religion impact on human health. That such a connection exists, and has been documented empirically, by this point cannot be assailed. But all of us who care about this field are admittedly vulnerable to criticism that we have ignored our responsibility to connect our data to substantive, comprehensible, and recognizable features of normative religious belief and practice as experienced and sanctioned within the living faith traditions of our study subjects. Good science is about more than describing and analyzing; it is also about explaining and interpreting. We have done an increasingly sophisticated job at the former, but a woefully marginal job at the latter.

All of us would benefit from taking a step back, to the early days of this field in the 1950s. The think-tank-style deliberations of the Academy of Religion and Mental Health are long gone, but our hope is that *Healing to All Their Flesh* will be a reasonable modern-day facsimile—the next best thing under the circumstances. The conversation begun (or, rather, renewed) in this book can give us some perspective as to where we should be going and why—perspective noticeably missing in most of the now thousands of published quantitative analyses. The substance of what this book has to offer can identify the ideas, concepts, and themes that we need to be engaging, and how, and ideally these can provide a sense of shared purpose and direction for this field.

This project is predicated on (and necessitated by) a very simple thesis: methodologically, on the one hand, studying the effects of religion may offer no uniquely intractable problems in comparison to any other domain of variables investigated in relation to health; but theoretically and conceptually, on the other hand, religion is quite unlike any of the other factors that are typically studied in relation to health. "Religion" is not a unitary garden-variety construct that can easily be operationalized, added to a survey or trial, plugged into a statistical model, and subjected to a generalizable conclusion. Actually, this *can* be done, and is, but often without the requisite reflection and understanding that makes results interpretable and meaningful in any coherent sense. A medical researcher would never conduct a study of the health impact of, say, environmental toxins or nutritional status or social support without first consulting an environmental toxicologist or a nutritionist or a sociologist who could expertly identify what questions to ask, what hypotheses to frame, and, once data were collected, how to analyze the data and then how to interpret findings. Yet, in studies of religion and health, this is done all the time; it is probably the norm. This is foolish, irresponsible, and self-defeating. How can one expect to intelligently investigate the influence of beliefs and practices related to expressions of religion without ever consulting experts on the study of religion? Or at least scholars whose job it is to know *something* about the topic. An MD degree or training as an epidemiologist, biomedical scientist, nurse, or clinical researcher by itself does not qualify one to conduct religious research.

The two editors of this book have begun to engage this subject, separately, in recent publications. One of us (J. L.), in an article published in the *Journal of Religion and Health* in 2009, has documented the considerable confusion throughout the research literature on religion and health with respect to conceptual definitions of religion, spirituality, and faith, on the one hand, and health, healing, medicine, and health care, on the other.[23] Coupled with an atheoretical approach to investigating interconnections between these groups of constructs, it is clear that this field is at a crossroads that will not be resolved simply with more data. The other of us (K. G. M.), in his book *Heal Thyself: Spirituality, Medicine, and the Distortion of Christianity*, coauthored with Dr. Joel James Shuman, has argued that the implicit presumptions of so much of the research in this field run counter to normative Christian understandings of the experience and ultimate meaning of sickness, health, and healing.[24] As a result, the research literature is founded on tacitly accepted religion-health connections that may present distorted expectations as to the instrumentality of personal and communal religious expression for the amelioration of human suffering.

There are common threads here: both of us, independently, have recognized that just as important as the methods used by investigators to produce data-based findings for this field are the underlying presumptions of what it is, precisely, that is being accomplished here and the motives and intentions underlying these presumptions. Why are we all doing this work, what do we expect to find, and do these expectations make sense? And how can we even begin to answer these questions without first identifying where we stand on important ontological and existential questions about human life and on the nature of the Divine and our relationship to It?

Healing to All Their Flesh is an effort to initiate systematic reflection on these and associated questions. This is a lot to tackle in one collection of essays. This is especially so when factoring in the diversity of perspectives within and among faith traditions, as well as the number of prominent faith traditions whose scholars have begun weighing in on this topic. We hope, then, that the present volume can be the first of what will become a series of discussions. The old Academy of Religion and Mental Health roundtables are truly missed; perhaps our book can pick up where that series left off.

We have begun with representative senior scholars from the religious traditions with which we are most familiar: Judaism and Christianity. We have invited comment from prominent theological, pastoral, ethical, and religious scholars from these two faiths—all of them individuals who have in the past written thoughtfully about the impact or implications of religion, broadly defined, on health, healing, medicine, or health care. We have given these individuals pretty much carte blanche to say whatever it is that they would like to say on this subject, guided by a few framing questions: Do canon or theology have anything to tell us about physical pathology and suffering, about healing and restoration? Are there implications from this for how religion, personally or communally experienced, might or should impact on health or on the delivery or use of health care? Is a potentially salutary function of faith or spirituality indeed consistent with the teachings of faith traditions? Is a more accurate or nuanced reading of what these traditions teach possible? Does the status of the human spirit really matter for the functioning and well-being of the body? Has this larger issue been misconstrued and misinterpreted in some ways, and if so how? What questions should we be asking instead—scientists and religious scholars alike—and where can we look for answers?

The result of these deliberations, we hope, is a provocative and engaging discussion of the how and why—and wherefore—of the interconnections among spirituality, theology, and health. Moreover, we also hope that this will become a primary text for the next generation of discourse in theology and medicine as well as for religion and health research. We would like to be able to look back at this project, some years in the future, and recognize *Healing to All Their Flesh* as a collection of thought-provoking essays that seeded many years of both theological scholarship and empirical study and served to advance our understanding of the meaning and implications of a continued rapprochement between spirituality and health. If this would come to pass, we would view our efforts as a success.

NOTES

1. Proverbs 4:20–22 (ESV).
2. Jeff Levin, *God, Faith, and Health: Exploring the Spirituality-Healing Connection* (New York: John Wiley & Sons, 2001); Harold G. Koenig, Dana E. King, and Verna Benner Carson, *Handbook of Religion and Health*, 2nd ed. (New York: Oxford University Press, 2012).
3. Jeff Levin and Harold G. Koenig, "Faith Matters: Reflections on the Life and Work of Dr. David B. Larson," in *Faith, Medicine, and Science: A Festschrift in Honor of Dr. David B. Larson*, ed. Jeff Levin and Harold G. Koenig (New York: Haworth Pastoral Press, 2005), 3–25.

4. Harold G. Koenig, Michael E. McCullough, and David B. Larson, *Handbook of Religion and Health* (New York: Oxford University Press, 2001).

5. Koenig, King, and Carson, *Handbook of Religion and Health*, 2nd ed.

6. William Osler, "The Faith that Heals," *British Medical Journal* 1 (1910): 1470–72.

7. John Shaw Billings, "Vital Statistics of the Jews," *North American Review* 153 (1891): 70–84.

8. Amariah Brigham, *Observations on the Influence of Religion upon the Health and Physical Welfare of Mankind* [1835] (New York: Arno Press, 1973).

9. Jeff Levin, "Esoteric Healing Traditions," *EXPLORE: The Journal of Science and Healing* 4 (2008): 101–12.

10. Thomas S. Kuhn, *The Structure of Scientific Revolutions*, 2nd ed. (Chicago: University of Chicago Press, 1970),

11. Academy of Religion and Mental Health, *Religion, Science, and Mental Health: Proceedings of the First Academy Symposium on Inter-discipline Responsibility for Mental Health—a Religious and Scientific Concern, 1957* (New York: New York University Press, 1959).

12. Academy of Religion and Mental Health, *Religion in the Developing Personality: Proceedings of the Second Academy Symposium, 1958* (New York: New York University Press, 1960).

13. Academy of Religion and Mental Health, *Religion, Culture, and Mental Health: Proceedings of the Third Academy Symposium, 1959* (New York: New York University Press, 1961).

14. Academy of Religion and Mental Health, *The Place of Value Systems in Medical Education: Fourth Academy Symposium of the Academy of Religion and Mental Health* (New York: Academy of Religion and Mental Health, 1961).

15. Academy of Religion and Mental Health, *Research in Religion and Health: Selected Projects and Methods: Proceedings of the Fifth Academy Symposium, 1961* (New York: Fordham University Press, 1963).

16. Academy of Religion and Mental Health, *Moral Values in Psychoanalysis: Proceedings of the Sixth Academy Symposium, 1963* (New York: Academy of Religion and Mental Health, 1965).

17. Levin, *God, Faith, and Health.*

18. Kenneth Vaux, "Religion and Health," *Preventive Medicine* 5 (1976): 522–36, quotation on p. 522.

19. Harold Y. Vanderpool, "Is Religion Therapeutically Significant?" *Journal of Religion and Health* 16 (1977): 255–59, quotation on p. 256.

20. Berton H. Kaplan, "A Note on Religious Beliefs and Coronary Heart Disease," *Journal of the South Carolina Medical Association* 15 (5 Suppl.) (1976): 60–64.

21. Paul Tillich, *The Meaning of Health: The Relation of Religion and Health*, ed. Paul Lee (Richmond, CA: North Atlantic Books, 1981).

22. Peter H. Van Ness, "Theology and Epidemiology as Complementary Perspectives on Aging," *Journal of Religious Gerontology* 15 (2003): 25–40.

23. Jeff Levin, "'And Let Us Make Us a Name': Reflections on the Future of the Religion and Health Field," *Journal of Religion and Health* 48 (2009): 125–45.

24. Joel James Shuman and Keith G. Meador, *Heal Thyself: Spirituality, Medicine, and the Distortion of Christianity* (New York: Oxford University Press, 2003).

PART 1

JEWISH PERSPECTIVES

THE CHAPTERS in this first section of *Healing to All Their Flesh* approach the interface of Judaism with health, healing, and medicine from a diversity of perspectives, emphasizing varied themes. Their rabbinic authors, as a whole, represent multiple denominational streams, including Reform, Reconstructionist, and Conservative Judaism. Still, common emphases are present, indicative of how a characteristically rabbinic approach to the subject of religion and health is fundamentally distinct from how Christian theologians, across the Christian spectrum, might choose to engage it.

Bill Cutter's reflective and very personal essay draws on his own experiences many years ago in the patient role, interpreting what he went through in light of contemporary rabbinic and Jewish medical discourse on the body, on Jewish law, and on ethics and values, and of Rabbi Levi Meier's writings on humanistic medicine. Richie Address provides a provocative take on critical existential issues, including regarding technology, autonomy, and spirituality, that arise in the lives of aging baby boomers as they begin to confront the limits of longevity and to negotiate issues of meaning. Dayle Friedman also explores aging, from a uniquely kabbalistic perspective, proposing Lifespan Judaism as a framework for older Jews experiencing both the losses and the opportunities for redemption that characterize the spiritual journey into old age. Elliot Dorff has crafted a comprehensive statement on how we can engage the *halakhic* (Jewish-legal) process in order to respond to contemporary bioethical challenges that may newly arise while remaining true to traditional Jewish perspectives on moral decision making. Simkha Weintraub's warm and hopeful message is at once a lucid and depthful meditation on healing and healers, grounded in the rabbinic literature, and also a thoughtful guide for future scholarship on Jewish healing.

Throughout these chapters, the contributors draw on the body of rabbinic writing to develop original approaches to pressing issues: the experience of patienthood and of aging, the need to make medical decisions that are consistent with Jewish moral guidance, and the innate longing of all Jews for healing experiences that are honoring of a uniquely Jewish spirituality. This emphasis on turning to the rabbis—to Mishnah, Talmud, and Midrash; to the *responsa* literature; to *kabbalah* and *mussar*; to creative contemporary writings—underscores a reverent valuation of the works of those who have come before, who have struggled with the same issues and efforted to reason through them in a way that is consistent with the teachings of the Torah that God gave to Moses. This approach characterizes rabbinic methodology and richly informs these chapters.

WILLIAM CUTTER

1. CURE AND HEALING, WHERE GOD MET SCIENCE

Four Decades of Spiritual Progress

My religious journey in the world of health and healing has included taking care of other people, while paying attention to my own sometimes failing body. It had a lot to do with all of the bodies that make up what we call society. The journey began nearly thirty-five years ago when a young Orthodox rabbi visited me during the first of several lengthy hospitalizations, and features—in his efforts at *bikkur cholim*—some annoying but important religious questions. In 1978, I was already a fairly well-established administrator and junior faculty member at Hebrew Union College in Los Angeles, a husband of just a few years, and the father of a three-year-old boy. I was surely more worldly than the young rabbi, and a bit more polished professionally. But he was bolder and more straightforward in that naïve way that some good people have when they innocently enter worlds new and strange. I suppose the politeness of my Midwestern upbringing and the rigorous intellectualism of my college education were responsible for my perfunctory management of "spirituality," and a little jolt of straightforward candor helped a lot. The young Orthodox rabbi was Levi Meier—a *yeshiva* graduate with ambitions to gain a PhD in psychology, and with intentions—to be fulfilled quite handsomely over the years—to remain a hospital rabbi who could draw on the deepest mysteries of the soul through religious faith and a slightly Jungian psychological tradition. (That tradition gets discussed somewhat in the new film *A Dangerous Method*.)

Rabbi Meier depended upon religious archetypes for his understanding of illness and human fragility, and he located some of these ancient patterns within Jewish classic texts. He shared his beliefs implicitly with all of his patients, and explicitly and intellectually with those whom he felt could understand his particular philosophical blendings. They were foreign to most of his Orthodox religious colleagues, while his religious view was foreign to many of his patients at the medical center.

In that early visit, Rabbi Meier asked me simply what God had to do with my recovery. I was shocked by the question and responded rapidly that this was "something I had to think about"; but I was surprisingly propelled into a thirty-five-year effort to answer the question. What follows here is some description of the journey that began that morning at Cedars-Sinai Medical Center, a large and powerful institution that somehow made way for the intimate journeys of vulnerable individuals. It is a journey that, to some extent, traces the "progress" of three decades and more that have transpired since that simple but fateful morning as I lay exposed to a thousand medical interventions, and only one self named Bill Cutter who presumably believed in one God. Adding to Rabbi Meier's part in the undoing of my spiritual apathy is material that he himself gathered from leading thinkers of his time—and which he published at the end of the next decade.[1]

We have come through a lot of changes in the world of healing since hospitals throughout America began to think about the role of formalized spiritual attention to the patients who are being patched, detoxified, and rearranged. To assist in all of this medical work, an entire pastoral movement has sprung up with its own rules for qualification and its own goals and objectives. I have been involved in that movement almost since its beginning and have watched it formalize to a sometimes exaggerated degree.

I hope that readers of the collection of essays before us may be interested in at least one person's view of the changes that have occurred over thirty-plus years—both within the life of one man, and within the general spiritual discourse that has been the cause and perhaps the result of my journey. (I suggest with some pride, that perhaps I have helped some of the changes along through programs that have been sponsored by my institution's Kalsman Institute on Judaism and Health.)

Levi Meier's innocent question to me in 1978 occurred at the beginning of his own effort to explore the healing value of the sick room visit, the religious meaning of lending a hand, and his effort to help people understand what they were experiencing as caregivers and care receivers. The floors of Cedars-Sinai have never been the same. Since Rabbi Meier began scurrying around those floors at breakneck speed, counseling countless volunteers who worked under his guidance, organizing programs with his loyal assistant, Paula Ven Gelder, and corralling young *yeshiva* children who bring *shabbos* (the Sabbath) into the hospital on Friday afternoons, Cedars-Sinai has entered into a grand plan of pastoral care to accompany its significant clinical contribution to the health of Los Angeles.

When Levi Meier first conceived the idea for his book *Jewish Values in Health and Medicine*,[2] he was trying to conceptualize the relationship between the patient's experience of illness and some of the health issues that were surfacing among Jews who cared about what our tradition had to offer. He seemed, I now see in retrospect, to be drawing upon an ancient Talmudic story in which only the proffered hand is able to elevate the ill person.[3] His book was a decidedly humanistic effort—a way of looking at the "whole" of health delivery and the effect of that delivery on those who received it—but humanistic attached to a religious spirit. He was not the first to think in terms of this kind of humanistic medicine, but he was among the most insistent, and his book managed to bring together some fine Jewish scientific minds and learned religious leaders with the experience of patients who had benefited from that science and yet longed for Jewish inspiration beyond physical cure: a young woman who suffered early nearly fatal heart disease; a prominent and revered rabbi whose experience with bypass surgery was laden with Jewish reflection; a younger rabbi (me) who was determined to relate the writing life to the experiencing life. It was a unique gathering.

Of course there was a Jewish tradition that had addressed health and healing: Maimonides, and a few other classic Jewish medical figures (Assaf, for example) who provided principles and expectations for the healer's role. Modern exemplars—like some of the authors in this book—had begun to think about medical ethics and Jewish responsibility. In the general domain, there was already a highly developed complementary medicine industry, and there had always been food advocates like Adele Davis and religious "outliers" like Christian and Jewish Scientists, homeopaths, and California optimists. But the mainstreaming of notions about spirit and body had not yet occurred, and no system for extraclinical healing was even being discussed; and men and women like Levi Meier pushed forward an agenda that by 2012 has come to dominate the health pages of daily newspapers, even as it has become the subject of countless essays in medical journals and conferences that are devoted to the healing that can lie behind cure. Of that distinction I shall speak further on, but surely the present volume you are now reading is a stunning example of that mainstreaming.

There is a kind of prescience to Rabbi Meier's seemingly innocent collection of essays: a discussion of human dignity by Rabbi David Hartman,[4] who has by now become legendary in the liberal Jewish communities of America by virtue of his entrepreneurship and his willingness to look at religious issues in new ways; an article by the significant Rabbi-physician Fred Rosner on the patient-physician relationship;[5] Dr. Rosner's reflections on how we as Jews must handle the AIDS epidemic from a moral and public policy point of view;[6] and ethical reflections by the prominent Los Angeles neurosurgeon, Dr. Milton Heifetz.[7]

One of the most stimulating discussions in the entire book is represented by two essays on end-of-life care, and the emergence of hospice as a healing entity in Jewish life. It is a kind of dialogue between two major figures in American Orthodoxy. In that regard, the book represents an archival resource on one of modernity's most interesting problems: How can the Jewish notion of "every moment of life being of infinite value" be harmonized with the reality of end-of-life costs to society, and the suffering that is probably extended for patients and family through the endless interventions that now—in the shadow of futility—can prolong a life beyond reasonable term. The dialogue—implied only—between Rabbi Maurice Lamm[8] and Rabbi J. David Bleich[9] in just this regard elevates *Jewish Values in Health and Medicine* to an essential document of its time and establishes the book as a harbinger of one of modernity's key dilemmas. Rabbi Bleich's conclusion regarding the establishment of hospice as being problematic—however well-intentioned—and Rabbi Lamm's more existential and narrative way of looking at the issue are "tropes," if you will, of Jewish thinking around a variety of issues in ethics and talmudic-*halakhic* discourse. When can one draw upon the existential experience of individuals to influence an entire value system?!

So using Rabbi Meier's book as a touchstone for examining the progress that we have made over three decades, one sees that large issues like the presence of AIDS in the Jewish community, the way in which we have to handle end-of-life care, and our understanding of surrogate parenthood have blossomed into major questions that are not only still with us, but have become elaborated with new implications in our increasingly complex society and because of our increasingly problematic economic environment. The more intimate issues like patient autonomy, the struggle to find hope in the hospital room, and the companionship that seems to be swiftly disappearing from the doctor-patient relationship, continue to take on implications and to require the spiritual probing that have been exhibited in the diaries and poems of some of our great writers, and in the struggles of spiritual leadership to assist people on their healing journeys.

Which leads me back to Rabbi Meier's question: What had God to do with my recovery in 1978–79? First, of course, came the repair of heart muscle, the opening of vessels, the gaining of physical strength.

The bills paid, some perspective gained, and a strategy for finding a parking place at the hospital's rehabilitation center finally calculated, my spiritual journey could begin.

I conclude my own essay by citing another written by Dr. Jerome Groopman, legendary Boston physician and writer, in *The New Yorker* over a decade ago.[10] "God on the Brain" exposed Dr. Groopman's management of the sometimes disruptive gap between faith and science. It is an essay that probably would not have been published much earlier than the 1990s, by which time the American public was more curious about matters of the spirit. For *The New Yorker*'s audience, it was a rare event, in any case. Here was a modern physician, a man of science, evidence, and action, facing a probably nonreligious audience, writing about his own attachment to the ancient religions of the Jewish people. The essay makes it clear that Dr. Groopman does not see faith as involving praying to God to make one person well, but—rather—sees religious relevance through a much more complex set of values. The man who has contributed so much to the clinical well-being of thousands of sufferers actually prays in the morning in defiance of the science that has sometimes distanced human beings from God as well as from other human beings. Lewis Thomas observed years ago that technological innovations have improved our science but too often put a piece of equipment between doctor and patient.[11] For me, part of that lost intimacy between doctor and patient has to do with God in the hospital room. For Dr. Groopman, the great intellectual traditions of Judaism joined with the more intimate and ambiguous spirituality of the Carpathian Mountains to create a great physician and a spiritual devotee.

My essay—less eloquent perhaps than Dr. Groopman's—reflects the inspiration of science and faith that has animated most of my life these past three-plus decades. It probably would not have been of much interest in the middle of the last century, as we were riding high on the waves of medical and surgical progress and most of us seemed more perfunctory in our performance of religious duty—if we performed it at all. My small contribution to Rabbi Meier's early book on Jewish values and medicine[12] turns out to be one among thousands of writings that—I propose—have helped make the current health climate more hospitable to spiritual probings. The change in the way we talk about religion and health has come from some of the changes that enabled Dr. Groopman's writing in his essay on God, and my personal experience with doctoring, my own body, and the Jewish world that I inhabit has demonstrated to me that the individual body can only be understood as part of the body politic—sorely in need of healing to be sure.

My notion of "body politic" has to do with the sum of human experience—an ennobling of our physical existence into the status of spiritual entity. It draws on some of the recent theological thinking of Arthur Green, whose recent book *Radical Judaism*[13] argues that God may exist in horizontal space rather than at some vertical remove. My own convictions draw heavily on the idea that God is the representation of the maximum of human experience—barely imagined, and yet experienced implicitly day to day. I think it is especially beholden to the perspectives of the nineteenth-century social scientist Emile Durkheim, the brilliant heir to rabbis who eschewed his rabbinic patrimony but clung to a kind of theology that I hold out to physicians and to others in the healing profession. (As an aside, I once wrote to my twelve physicians that they could try a little theology to go with their cardiology, urology, oncology, and pathology.) Durkheim wrote this thought early in his intellectual life, to paraphrase: "Society is the 'real' object to which the word 'God' points."[14]

Robert Bellah, one of Durkheim's heirs, has reminded us that the French thinker did not idolize society as some have thought, but actually meant (only) to deepen the word "society" so that it could take the place of the "great word it supersedes."[15] Divinity, then, becomes part of the essence of society, and it is in that spirit that I bring poems to health professionals, urge a kind of presence upon my students when they visit ill people, and ask practitioners and their institutions to move beyond the immediate care they are providing with the experience of the totality of purpose that lies behind every effort to make someone feel better. My favorite tool is poetry, that great vehicle that surprises with every rhythm shift and metaphoric idea, but others have found their tools as well in prayer and meditation, and even in simple conversational relationship.

We have experienced stunning developments in our definitions of healing since the appearance of Levi Meier's first book. We now talk matter-of-factly about the difference between healing and curing (see my own book, *Midrash and Medicine*[16]). But we also have encountered new and complex economic problems, we have become aware of epidemics in parts of the world that were once hidden from our eyes, and the entire medical environment today seems worlds away from where it was when I first became a patient: more quantified and less reliable at the same time. We have seen that some of the ethical methodologies on which we have drawn do not suit our new economic and technological age. There are hopeful signs: this very consciousness of our crises will someday bear new spiritual fruit; groups of people take ethical probing ever more seriously in hospitals; women have added new interpersonal dimensions to doctoring; and our science continues to bring some promise.

Our progress, both technologically and spiritually, has come at some price. It would seem that patient autonomy has helped ill individuals take more responsibility for their healing, but it also has made doctoring inconvenient for some doctors; the notion that life is of infinite value will clash with the reality that life might also have infinite cost; our communities will have to reorganize to take care of a swiftly aging population; and the way we organize life for the fragile and needy will have to change. I see a change occurring among those of us who are asking new questions of old texts; we shall probably no longer be satisfied with looking for normative guidance from our classics, but we should seek out, rather, a community-building effort through attachment to heritage. Durkheim's community will be the source of our strength in finitude; but as that strength expands, it may help people reach beyond their finitude into aspirations for holiness. And imaginative definitions of what "God" means will make it possible for a more open discourse of healing in a world sadly in need of repair.

NOTES

1. Levi Meier, *Jewish Values in Psychotherapy: Essays on Vital Issues on the Search for Meaning* (Lanham, MD: University Press of America, 1988).
2. Levi Meier, ed., *Jewish Values in Health and Medicine* (Lanham, MD: University Press of America, 1991).
3. *Berachot* 5b.
4. David Hartman, "Human Dignity as Reflected in the Physician-Patient Relationship: A Philosophical Jewish Perspective," in Meier, *Jewish Values in Health and Medicine*, 81–94.
5. Fred Rosner, "The Patient-Physician Relationship: Responsibilities and Limitations," in Meier, *Jewish Values in Health and Medicine*, 95–112.
6. Fred Rosner, "The Acquired Immunodeficiency Syndrome (AIDS): Jewish Perspectives," in Meier, *Jewish Values in Health and Medicine*, 171–84.
7. Milton Heifetz, "A Concept of Ethics," in Meier, *Jewish Values in Health and Medicine*, 73–79.
8. Maurice Lamm, "The Jewish Way in Dying: The Jewish Component in Hospice Care," in Meier, *Jewish Values in Health and Medicine*, 113–25.
9. J. David Bleich, "Care of the Terminally Ill," in Meier, *Jewish Values in Health and Medicine*, 141–61.
10. Jerome Groopman, "God on the Brain: The Curious Coupling of Science and Religion," *The New Yorker* (September 17, 2001): 165–68.
11. Lewis Thomas, "The Technology of Medicine," in *The Lives of a Cell: Notes of a Biology Watcher* (New York: Viking Press, 1974), 31–36.
12. William Cutter, "Growing Sick: Thoughts on Months as a Heart Patient, Years as a Rabbi," in Meier, *Jewish Values in Health and Medicine*, 29–40.
13. Arthur Green, *Radical Judaism: Rethinking God and Tradition* (New Haven, CT: Yale University Press, 2010).
14. Paraphrased by Robert N. Bellah, "Introduction," in *Emile Durkheim: On Morality and Society*, ed. Robert N. Bellah (Chicago: University of Chicago Press, 1973), ix–lv, quotation on p. ix.
15. Bellah, "Introduction," x.
16. William Cutter, ed., *Midrash and Medicine: Healing Body and Soul in the Jewish Interpretive Tradition* (Woodstock, VT: Jewish Lights, 2011).

RICHARD ADDRESS

2. CONTEMPLATING A THEOLOGY OF HEALTHY AGING

It is a wonderful custom, at times of celebration, to raise a glass and drink *l'chaim,* to life. It is an honored tradition to wish someone on their birthday, to live *ad meah v'esrim*, to one hundred and twenty, channeling Moses' life span from the book of Deuteronomy. The celebration and honoring of life is a basic part of the Jewish tradition, regardless of one's denominational affiliation. Implicit, however, in the toasts and wishes is a life of health and wellness. The challenges of longevity and the attendant progress and impact of medical technology has provided the contemporary Jewish community with new challenges and understandings as to what that "life" can or should be. We wish for long life with health and the mental acuity to enjoy that life; we do not wish to have that life lived in illness, in disease, or in an isolated existence in which our mental abilities have been stripped by dementia or Alzheimer's. Health and wellness are the real wish and point of many prayers and rituals. The theological questions of meaning and purpose that are allied with issues of health and wellness have become increasingly present within the Jewish community. Medical technology has given us the gift of longevity and with the science often comes the religious question of "what for?" Imbedded in the linkage of modern medicine and Jewish tradition are the basic "why" questions that leap from Genesis 3 in which the issue of mortality is raised and in which God asks the basic question of human existence: *Ayecha? Where are you?* We spend our lives seeking an answer to that question and in doing so each of us confronts the fundamental questions of our own existence: Why was I born? Why must I die? What is the purpose for my being?

JUDAISM AND MEDICINE

The link between Judaism and medicine can be traced back to biblical times. It has undergone changes as Judaism has evolved and changed, and that linkage has often reflected the times and locations in which various Jewish communities were living. Health and wellness are to be prized and the care of the body is a reflection of our relationship with God. This is a basic principle of Judaism and is reflected in the following classic *midrash* or parable drawn from rabbinic tradition:

A story is told of Hillel that when he finished a lesson with his pupils, he accompanied them from the classroom. They said: "Master, where are you going?" Hillel replied: "To perform a religious duty." "Which duty is that?" they asked. "To bathe in the bathhouse," answered Hillel. The students asked: "Is this a religious obligation?" Hillel replied: "If someone is appointed to scrape and clean the statues of the king that are set up in the theatres and circuses and is paid to do the work, and furthermore, associates with the nobility, how much the more should I, who am created in the divine image and likeness, take care of my body?"[1]

We are created in the divine image and thus are bidden to care for the body as a reflection of the primary relationship between man and God. This is basic Jewish thought. In order to make sure this body is cared for properly, we must be mindful of our physical, emotional, and spiritual health. This holistic approach, basic I believe to a Jewish approach to health and wellness, finds its way even into prayers. Daily a Jew prays for healing and gives thanks that the finely balanced network of veins and arteries is working as it should, lest we would be unable to stand before God. This beautiful piece of liturgy is found in the morning service:

Blessed is Adonai our God, Sovereign of the universe.
With divine wisdom You have made our bodies,
combining veins, arteries and vital organs

into a finely balanced network.
Wondrous Maker and Sustainer of life,
were one of these to fail—how well we are aware!—
we would lack the strength to stand in life before You.
Blessed are You, Adonai,
Source of our health and strength.[2]

The theology is plain and direct. God has created us in a divine image. Our bodies, and life, are a gift and we are bidden to care for them in order that we may "stand in life" before God.

In the Bible, we have many instances of someone appealing directly to God to heal a person who has become ill. One of the most famous of these is the prayer spoken by Moses asking God to heal his sister Miriam. He pleads to God, "O God, pray heal her!"[3] Tradition accounts this as the first healing prayer in Jewish tradition and it has found its way back into contemporary usage as part of healing services or as a melody that accompanies special prayers for healing that are now part of many synagogue worship services. The prayer also sees the use of the Hebrew term for heal, *r'pha,* which evolves into the word for physician, *ropheh,* meaning "healer." This very direct approach was not always so. Biblical texts are filled with instances of divination and assorted other methods that were seen to provide healing and wellness. Despite injunctions in the Torah against consulting sorcerers and diviners, "healing practices involving magical spells, incantations, and exorcisms had found considerable expression. This was especially true in those Jewish communities influenced by Egyptian, Midianite, or Roman culture as Numbers, Isaiah, 2 Chronicles, Ezekiel, and 2 Kings attest."[4] The impact of various cultures and the lack of a binding and enforceable religious authority in postbiblical times "witnessed an increase in the use of various healing remedies, including exorcism of demons and the use of amulets."[5] This tradition carried on throughout the rabbinic period and, truth be told, remnants of many of these beliefs and practices still can be found today in family traditions and superstitions. This diversity in approach to healing, health, and responses to illness reflect the historical truth that there is no singular Jewish dogma for healing, no one set of prayers or practice, and no simple intellectual constructs to help us heal. Jewish thought from each period has bequeathed a different mode of alleviating suffering, and Jews from every subsequent period have added or enhanced some elements of healing, de-emphasized others, and borrowed ideas from contemporary non-Jewish sources.... Perhaps the most fundamental commonalities are a search for God, a reverence for life, a belief in the sacredness of heath, and a life-defining conviction that illness is an evil to be banished.[6]

At the root of all of these exhortations, edicts, and interpretations is the fundamental understanding that we are to take care of our health and bodies and life so as to be able to be in relationship with God. Thus, it is not surprising that Judaism established a special place for those individuals who became healers, or physicians. One of the earliest examples of this can be found in the writings of Ben Sira:

> Make friends with the physician, for he is essential to you;
> him also God has established in his profession.
> From God the doctor has his wisdom,
> and from the king he receives his sustenance.
> Knowledge makes the doctor distinguished
> and gives him access to those in authority.
> God makes the earth yield healing herbs,
> which the prudent should not neglect.
> Was not the water sweetened by a twig
> that people may learn its power?
> He endows humans with the knowledge
> to glory in his mighty works
> Through which the doctor eases pain
> and the druggist prepares his medicines;
> Thus God's creative work continues without cease
> in its efficacy on the surface of the earth.
> My son when you are ill, delay not,
> but pray to God, for it is he who heals.
> Flee wickedness; purify your hands,
> cleanse your heart of every sin.
> Offer your sweet smelling oblation and memorial,

a generous offering according to your means.
Then give the doctor his place
lest he leave, for you need him too,
There are times that give him an advantage,
and he too beseeches God
That his diagnosis may be correct
and his treatment bring about cure.
Whoever is a sinner toward his Maker
will be defiant toward the doctor.[7]

Again the theological position of Judaism is clear. The fundamental relationship we have is with God, and it is God who endows the physician the power to heal. This linkage and ability to heal were established through the interpretation of texts by rabbis. Everything within Jewish tradition, up to the present, is based on textual analyses and interpretation. Several texts from the Torah have been used to give scriptural validity, and thus authority, to allow humans to try to stop illness and heal. Two passages in Exodus were seen to mean that we have permission to heal. In Exodus 15:26, God promises that if the Israelites heed God and do what is right, he will not bring upon them the diseases visited upon the Egyptians because "I am the Lord your healer." Again, the Hebrew root of "your healer" is *resh, fey, aleph,* which is the root also for the noun "healer" or physician. Likewise in Exodus 21:19, we have the same root repeated in the context of verses that deal with monetary compensation for a victim of a fight. The repetition of the word has been interpreted to underscore the importance of causing someone to be healed. The classic text in Leviticus 19:16 which says that we are "not to stand idly by the blood of one's kinsman" was also interpreted as a mandate to allow human beings to heal. The obligation of the healer "to not stand idly by" was echoed in the classic sixteenth-century code *Shulchan Aruch*: "The Torah gave permission to the physician to heal; moreover this is a religious precept and is included in the category of saving life; and if he withholds his services, it is considered as shedding blood."[8]

Another of the major texts that has been used to reinforce the need to restore health to a sick person can be seen in Deuteronomy 22:1–2. The biblical text reads as follows: "If you see your fellow's ox or sheep gone astray, do not ignore it; you must take it back to your fellow. If your fellow does not live near you or you do not know who he is, you shall bring it home and it shall remain with you until your fellow claims it; then you shall give it back to him." Some translations of the last part of this section translate the Hebrew *v'ha'sha'voto lo,* as "and you shall restore it to him." Maimonides sees in this verse a clear mandate to interrupt nature, for he reasons that when one is sick, one has lost one's health (and thus one's ability to be in a healthy relationship with God) and therefore it is mandatory for the physician to restore to the individual his/her health. As he wrote in his commentary to the *Mishnah Nedarim* 4:4: "It is obligatory from the Torah for the physician to heal the sick, and this obligation is included in the explanation of the scriptural phrase *and you shall restore it to him*, meaning to heal his body."[9]

The role of the physician as enabler of God's work finds its way through Jewish history in a variety of instances. Typical is the following *midrash*, which tells of the time when Rabbis Ishmael and Akiba were walking through the streets of Jerusalem and came upon a man who was sick. The sick person turned to the rabbis and asked: "How can I be cured?" The rabbis replied that he should just do such and such until he was cured. "But who afflicted me?" asked the sick person. "The Holy One, blessed be He," responded the rabbis. The stranger then asked: "So how can you interfere in a matter that is not your concern? God afflicted me and you wish to heal?" Ishmael and Akiba then asked: "What is your profession?" "I am a tiller of the soil. Here is the vine cutter in my hand." "But who created the vine?" asked the rabbis. "The Holy One, blessed be He," replied the man. Akiba and Ishmael responded: "Well, you interfered in a vineyard which was not yours. God created it and you cut away its fruits?" The man answered back: "But were I not to plow and till and fertilize and weed, the vineyard would not produce any fruit." The rabbis responded: "So, from your own work have you not learned what is written 'as for man his days are like grass' (Psalm 103:15). Just as the tree, if not weeded, fertilized and plowed, will not grow and bring forth its fruits, so with the human body. The fertilizer is the medicine and the means of healing, and the tiller of the earth is the healer."[10]

Likewise, we have instances of prayers and oaths from Jewish physicians from centuries ago that also reflected the understanding that the doctor was doing God's work and that ultimately all healing came from God, who placed the ability to heal in the hands of the doctor. Asaph wrote such an oath to his disciples that is framed by the author's understanding that being mindful of God and following God's commandments will be the foundation for their ability to treat patients.[11] One of the most famous of these prayers was attributed to Maimonides (twelfth century), but in reality was authored, according to some, by Marcus Herz, an eighteenth-century German physician:

> Almighty God, Thou has created the human body with infinite wisdom. . . . Thou has endowed man with the wisdom to relieve the suffering of his brother, to recognize his disorders, to extract the healing substances, to discover their powers and to prepare and to apply them to suit every ill. In thine Eternal Providence Thou hast chosen me to watch over the life and health of Thy creatures. I am now about to apply myself to the duties of my profession. Support me, Almighty God, in these great labors, that they may benefit mankind, for without Thy help not even the least thing will succeed.[12]

The prayer goes on to ask for guidance from God and that his patients have trust in his decisions. The author asks that he have patience and calm and that he also may have the ability to learn from others who may have more knowledge than he in a specific situation. Again, the prayer is instructive as it continues the thread of the relationship between the physician and God.

There is a sense of partnership between the doctor and God within classic Jewish tradition. This partnership carries over even to today, perhaps couched differently, as evidenced by the great twentieth-century theologian Rabbi Abraham Joshua Heschel. I suggest that the renewed interest in health, healing, and Jewish tradition can be traced to a speech Heschel gave in 1964 before the American Medical

Association entitled "The Patient as a Person." Heschel reflected Jewish tradition in outlining the sacred partnership between science and the spirit and between doctor and patient in the task of healing. "The doctor," wrote Heschel, "is God's partner in the struggle between life and death. Religion is medicine in the form of a prayer; medicine is prayer in the form of a deed. . . . It is a grievous mistake to keep a wall of separation between medicine and religion. There is a division of labor but a unity of spirit. The act of healing is the highest form of *imitatio Dei*. To minister to the sick is to minister to God. Religion is not the assistant of medicine but the secret of one's passion for medicine."[13]

Heschel reminds us of the sacred relationship that exists between the physician and the patient, a relationship that models the ideal relationship between God and mankind. The interest in a more "holistic" approach to medicine and the doctor-patient relationship that seems to many so "new," is, I suggest, a reflection of traditional Jewish thought. Everything in the universe is interconnected and the intersection of the mind, body, and spirit is a natural part of how Judaism and Jewish tradition looks at healing and wellness.

The "new age" approach to healing is not so new after all. For example, Dr. Andrew Weil, an exemplar of this more holistic approach to health, may have been channeling his inner Maimonides when he wrote: "In taking a history from a new patient, I ask many questions about lifestyle, about relationships, hobbies, ways of relaxing, patterns of eating and exercising, sex and spiritual interests."[14] Writing in the twelfth century, the scholar-physician Maimonides outlined his approach, as noted by contemporary scholar Dr. Mordechai Reich:

> First, the physician needs to obtain a clear understanding of the patient's subjective world and secure a diagnosis of the patient's psychological distress. Even if psychological stress is not manifest, it is assumed to exist, and the physician is required to search for it. Only after this "psychological workup" can the physician begin with a medical intervention. Of the patient, Maimonides demands a willingness to undertake an introspective process and adhere strictly to the regimen that the physician would formulate. Once the patient and the physician embark on a carefully directed program which

includes an examination of thoughts, feelings, and philosophy of life, as well as any necessary medical interventions, a partial or total cure is likely. Maimonides expects that the patient's "spirits would be raised and depressive and self-defeating thoughts would decrease in frequency and vanish."[15]

THE APPLICATION OF A FUNDAMENTAL ETHIC TO DECISION MAKING

Jewish tradition understands that our bodies are gifts from God, that we treasure and promote health so we can best model our relationship with God, and that the physician is the primary actor in helping us maintain that relationship. We are bidden to have our health restored if we lose it, and our health is a composite of the interactions of mind, body, and spirit. If we could reduce all the texts and commentaries to a single fundamental ethic, I suggest that it would be the dignity and sanctity of human life and the preservation of that human life in dignity and sanctity. I believe that this principle correctly summarizes the various aspects of Jewish thought as it relates to issues of health and wellness, illness and healing. Our challenge in the modern world is to see how this fundamental principle applies to the real world. For in our day-to-day life we understand that decisions are rarely as clear-cut when it comes to issues of medicine, health, and healing. Often we are faced with decisions that challenge our own sense of ethics. In confronting the challenges of today, let me suggest that there are three "wild cards" that impact how we apply that principle to our lives. These three wild cards speak to where the contemporary Jewish community rests, especially the community in North America. The three "wild cards" that I refer to are technology, autonomy, and spirituality. They each play a part in how one makes a decision and how one looks at life and one's place in it. They each, eventually, help a person return to the fundamental questions of existence: Why was I born? Why must I die? Why, for what purpose, do I exist?

There should be in every prayer book a blessing that gives thanks for the miracles of medical technology. The progress and impact of this technology has literally reshaped life as we know it. Thanks to this technology people today are cruising the seas or back working at their jobs where years ago we would have attended their funerals. Thanks to this technology there are countless people, many we know, who are living productive lives with a disease that years ago would have been fatal. The science of medicine has produced what can only be called modern miracles. Yet, there remain, often in silence, the spiritual questions that have evolved as a result of these medical miracles. These are questions that spring from Job and Ecclesiastes; questions such as, "Why me?" "For what reason have I survived this cancer?" or, "Why am I still alive when my friend is not?"

Technology also has led to discussions regarding limits. Just because we can do something does not necessarily mean that we must. These questions point to a lack in so many congregations and communities of regularly scheduled conversations and forums on how Jewish tradition and texts understand the use and impact of this technology. There rarely is one answer; rather, each case, as tradition counsels us, must be treated on its own. I believe that in issues of health, healing, and wellness, *context* is an essential component of how we decide what to do and when to do it. A simple formula for decision making that I have used starts with the naming of the value that underlies the case: from the saving of a life (issues of end-of-life care) to being "fruitful and multiplying" (issues related to birth and pregnancy). We apply that value to the case before us. We examine the texts and mood of Jewish tradition that apply to the case, keeping in mind the fundamental principle of the dignity and sanctity of human life and the preservation of human life in dignity and sanctity. This of course reinforces the contextual aspect of this formula for dignity and sanctity are subjective and made the more so by the impact of medical technology.

It is often in the midst of these discussions involving context that the other two wild cards come in to play. The issue of personal autonomy, the second wild card, is very much a part of who we are in the contemporary Jewish world. Despite the teaching of tradition, many people do not hold to the belief that their bodies are gifts from God and that there may be limits, according to Jewish tradition, as to what may be acceptable or even permissible. This is another reason for heightened education in this area, for Judaism has much to say about negotiating humane decisions in times of illness. The myth of control that so many harbor comes into conflict with the reality that we really do not control many of the major issues that impact our lives. It is how we choose to react to these random acts that often determine the type of person we become and the course of our own life. Autonomy is limited by context and our autonomy is impacted by the choices we make.

How we choose is also influenced by a third wild card: our own spiritual beliefs. Again, modern congregations spend precious little time in affording people the opportunity to explore their beliefs, especially in light of how those beliefs reflect issues of health and illness. We come again to issues that are very subjective, terribly personal, and often extremely contextual. My own sense of dignity and sanctity may be one way at one stage of life and may change as I enter a new stage of life. We are all dynamic individuals in which change, from our cells to our worldview, is constantly in motion. Judaism seems to each of us as evolving and dynamic reflections of the divine and, thus, what we believe and how those beliefs get put into practice are issues that must be accounted for when we are called upon to make decisions about our own life. Thus, it is through the application of a value to a context that is influenced by technology, autonomy, and spirituality that helps guide us to choose an appropriate path. In applying the fundamental principle of dignity and sanctity, we can make use of the formula of value-context-choice as influenced by the wild cards of technology, autonomy, and spirituality.

THE REVOLUTION IN LONGEVITY

These wild cards, and the reality of seeing things within their context, will become increasingly an important part of a major evolving reality within the contemporary Jewish community of North America. I speak of the explosion of older Jews and reality of the revolution in longevity that is now making itself felt in very real ways within our community. There is a growing emphasis within the institutional Jewish community on trying to win the hearts, minds, and wallets of the twenty- and thirty-year-olds, as well as renewed emphasis on the increasingly disenfranchised teenaged population. All this is well and good. Yet I feel it is a major mistake to ignore the growing and spiritually assertive and searching multigenerational cohort of the newly aging. The baby boom generation represents the most creative and spiritually challenging aspect of our community. They may not be "the future"; however, they are very much the "present" and the decisions that they make will help determine the type of community that their children and grandchildren inherit. We ignore their spiritual concerns at our own peril.

It is this generation that has driven the revolution that has seen the re-visioning and reinterpretation of ritual. It is this generation that has led the spiritual revolution that marks so much of contemporary Jewish life. Blessed with economic and social freedom and security, as well as the real potential for decades of post-child-rearing life, this is the generation that continues to raise questions of its own legacy, as well as those of meaning and purpose. The baby boom generation is also the first generation that *expects* longevity and thus is more attuned to and concerned with issues that impact its own health.

As mentioned above, there is a massive and important need for education as to how Jewish texts and traditions can guide, hold, and support people as they navigate difficult health-related issues. Too few of the current members of the Jewish community are aware of the important messages that the tradition has to offer in areas that will impact every member of our community. With increasing frequency, families are now having to negotiate how to make decisions about themselves and loved ones, all the while influenced by the wild cards of technology, autonomy, and spirituality. What does it mean to live and preserve our lives in dignity and sanctity? This fundamental principle gives rise to some of the issues that will touch on health and wellness within the coming decades.

One of the greatest challenges in the present and coming years will be the ethical and moral decisions dealing with caregiving. There always have been caregivers. However, the blessings of longevity and technology have produced what really is a new life stage within our world. The caregiver is a stage that can last not just months or years, but, for some, decades. It impacts family systems and the health and wellness of the caregiver. We have been given the gift of longevity, yet longevity without health may not be the idealized blessing we all crave. Is there a time when it is permissible to allow the flame of life to flicker out? When is it permissible, perhaps even necessary, to cede the care of a loved one to someone else; and in doing so, how do we deal with the psychospiritual emotions that accompany such a decision? When is "enough, enough"? Is there any meaning in one's pain and suffering?

Jewish tradition gives guidance to these issues in many texts from the rabbinic period through the present. The mood of the tradition is humane. It sees the context of a situation as being powerful and important. It even has developed categories of illness that impact how one *may* proceed—for example, the category of *goses*. This is a Jewish legal term that signifies a patient who is close to death. The Talmudic ideal was within three days. Yet medical technology has rendered the literal interpretation almost meaningless. Instead, we refer to a patient who is *goses* as one who is close to death, a person for whom the arsenal of medical technology has been exhausted and for whom comfort care, or palliative care, is the prescribed course. Up to that border, the tradition urges that we do everything we can to honor that fundamental principle of the dignity and sanctity of human life and the preservation of that human life in dignity and sanctity. Yet even the rabbis of old understood that there may come a time when continued intervention may actually do more harm than good. Every rabbi and clergy person has had to sit and guide a family through the difficult labyrinth of decisions at life's end. It is instructive and soul saving for some to know that the decisions they are making are within the confines of their faith tradition. As difficult as these decisions may be, the support of one's own tradition helps alleviate much of the residual guilt that often reaches into a person's soul. The need to educate people as to these traditions has never been greater as the engine of medical technology continues to drive forward. The importance of these issues is clearly seen in the fact that among the denominations of contemporary Judaism there is more agreement within these areas of decision making than on any other issue.

The allied concerns of organ donation and hospice care also find more agreement among the various streams of contemporary Judaism. An example of a typical institutional response to some of these issues can be found in "Compassionate and Comfort Care Decisions at the End of Life," an official resolution adopted by the general assembly of the North American Reform movement in 1995.[16] This resolution takes into consideration the realities of modern medical technology and its impact on people. The resolution states that we know that medical technology "may also unnaturally prolong the dying process" and that while Reform Judaism is on record (as is all Judaism) that under certain conditions people have the right to refuse aggressive treatment, "it is clear that not all needs are met by withholding or withdrawal of medical treatment at the end of life." The resolution affirms the traditional belief that there is no dignity or sanctity in undue pain and suffering and, under the value of *pikuach nefesh* (saving of life), asks that we "strive toward an achievable goal: to provide a quality of life that is at least tolerable for each one whose journey ends in pain and suffering." Thus, the movement affirmed a call for hospice care in stating, "By providing caring support for families and assisting in the development of hospices and similar environments where spiritual and physical needs are met, our congregations can help preserve the meaning and purpose of our lives as we approach the end of the journey."

One of the great challenges that inform much of these discussions on end-of-life health issues has to do with the reality of pain and suffering. Much has been written on this issue across denominational lines. It is safe to say that the mood of current communal thought takes into account the issue of one's "quality of life." This is part of the discussion around the context of a case and the particular circumstance of an individual. This is also why every aspect of the community favors advance directives for medical treatment and health care powers of attorney. Tradition understood that one who is enduring great pain and suffering may lose a sense of reality. The Jewish legal tradition of *responsa* is helpful in trying to untangle the various approaches to this issue.

Responsa is the simple act of someone asking a question of a recognized Jewish authority and that authority writing an answer to the particular question, tracing the answer through Jewish tradition in order to arrive at a conclusion that speaks to the current world in which the question was raised. This is an ongoing and organic process, and there have been many *responsa* written in recent years that reflect concerns about health, healing, illness, and wellness. One such *responsum*, "Relieving Pain of a Dying Patient," asks if it is permissible to give a larger than usual dosage of pain medication to a person who is suffering, even though that dosage may hasten the person's death. The person is *goses*, in his final stages of life and in "agony." The *responsum* traces issues related to pain and the theological concerns of why people may suffer. It concludes with the following that is reflective of modern Jewish thought and modern medical practice:

> In other words, we may take definite action to relieve pain, even if it is of some risk to the *chayei-sha-a,* the last hours. In fact, it is possible to reason as follows: It is true that the medicine to relieve his pain may weaken his heart, but does not the great pain itself weaken his heart? And: May it not be that relieving the pain may strengthen him more than the medicine might weaken him? At all events, it is a matter of judgment, and in general we may say that in order to relieve his pain, we may incur some risk as to his final hours.[17]

These caregiving issues also give rise to the need for discussion around how we come to understand the Fifth Commandment of "honoring father and mother." Three times does this commandment appear in the Torah; twice using the Hebrew word *kabed*, honor,[18] and once using the Hebrew *tira'oo*, fear or respect.[19] In Exodus and Deuteronomy, we are told to "honor our father and mother," while in Leviticus we are told to "fear or respect our mother and father." The difference in usage is explained by rabbis by saying that this is to teach that both must be treated equally.

This commandment takes on significant interpretation in the Talmudic tractate *Kiddushin* 31b–32a, in which the words are discussed and interpreted in a way that speaks to our issues in the twenty-first century. In discussing these two concepts of "honor" and "respect" (*kabed* and *tirah*), the rabbis remind us that in no way must the dignity and sense of self-respect of any human being, regardless of age, be diminished by anything we do. This goes back to that fundamental ethic of dignity and sanctity. It is the duty of adult children to protect the dignity of their parents. It is the duty of caregivers to protect the dignity of people that they care for. This is not a responsibility to be taken lightly, and given the increasingly high rate of caregiving now before us, this is a reality that carries great weight in our society.

Benjamin Freedman cites an approach that is again drawn from textual interpretation. He looks at Exodus 21:17, which states that "one who insults his father or mother shall be put to death." Freedman notes that this verse can be used to underscore a Jewish approach to dignity and, thus, to preventing indignity and humiliation:

> The connection between these two may seem obscure. In fact the concept of cursing and that of indignity are etymologically identical in Hebrew. The term for cursing, whose root is *KLL*, is a verbal form deriving from *KL*. *KL* itself means, literally, "light" in the sense of "lacking in weight." To *KLL* someone, therefore, means to treat that person "lightly," without dignity. "To curse," *KLL*, therefore, is, in Hebrew, the precise linguistic and conceptual antonym of the act of "honoring," *KBD*, the same term found in the Fifth Commandment, which, as we have seen, means literally to treat the person in a "weighty" manner.[20]

The Talmudic discussion in *Kiddushin* also asked the question, in regard to taking care of a parent, "Who pays?" This is not a question to be taken lightly. As more of our people deal with taking care of parents who are living longer, and living in a variety of situations and facilities, the issue of "who pays" can take on many interpretations. The tradition, in keeping with the idea of dignity and respect and honor, makes it clear that, if possible, a parent should be responsible for his or her own life and needs. Many of us are inclined, when going to the market for mom or dad, to pay for them. Many of us may be inclined to see an older person and feel that we need to shelter them from living life. To do so in excess, or to do so without knowledge of a context, may be to infantilize that person, thus reducing their dignity and sense of worth.

A Talmudic story is told of a man who would give his father plenty to eat and who was to inherit hell. Another man would put his father to work in a mill and is said to inherit Eden. How is this possible? The rabbinic interpretation of this lesson is that the first man, in totally assuming all responsibility for his able father, reduces his sense of dignity. The second man allows his father to continue to derive a sense of self-worth and dignity, placing him in a situation where he can contribute and be active; or, to put it in our idiom, allows him a reason to get up in the morning. How this sense of "who pays?" is also relevant to our lives is being lived by millions every day. The rabbis understood that adult children who are caregivers often "pay" with time. We drive our loved ones to a doctor and wait with them. We take them home, often stopping at the pharmacy to pick up that prescription or at the diner to share a meal. Time, which in our world is often more valuable than money, is often the currency of the caregiver. Dr. Michael Chernick gave an excellent summary of much of the Talmudic discussion on this issue when he wrote:

> Though two opinions regarding who bears financial responsibility for an aged parent appear in the Talmud, the generally accepted preference was for the parent to pay for his or her food and clothing needs. This ruling stood in conflict with an older tradition which stated that children must honor their parents by spending on them. In order to maintain harmony between the two positions, the later Talmudic teachers claimed that the child's financial outlay took the form of loss of work time and profits it might bring. The child, then, was expected to help feed and clothe that parent if it was necessary. The food and clothing, however, was paid for by the parent.[21]

What insights from the tradition can be helpful when situations of caregiving become too difficult for the caregiver and his or her family? This issue relates directly to one of the challenges of the revolution in longevity. With increased life spans we are witnessing a steady rise in incidents of dementia and Alzheimer's disease. Here the subjects of dignity and sanctity are put to a real test. Anyone who has to deal with or care for a loved one suffering from these conditions knows first-hand how the issue of one's dignity and sanctity become regular topics of conversation. Significant spiritual questions are often raised that test one's personal theology and which also may come into conflict with one's institutional or denominational theology. Phrases like "she has no quality of life" or "he would never want to live this way" or "that really is not my mother anymore" are frequently heard. The challenge of caregiving in these situations can strain an individual and a family system and create health issues for the caregiver. Clergy are often faced with a question from a congregant asking, "when does it become too much to take care of someone?"

Yet that same conversation often contains the achingly serious concern of "but how can I put my dad in a place like that?" Judaism seems to be clear in its mood that when the strains of caregiving present a threat to one's own health and to the health and stability of a family, then it may be of a higher value to cede care to a third party.

Chernick quotes a famous passage from Maimonides' *Mishneh Torah* which states that an adult child should try to deal with a parent who has become incompetent according to the condition of the parent. If, however, the condition of the person being cared for deteriorates to such an extent that it becomes very difficult to continue care, the child may cede care to a third party. Of course, this situation is not limited to a parent. We know of cases where this scenario is played out in regard to a spouse, a close relative, or even a child. Each is entitled to and deserving of his or her sense of dignity and respect; thus, when conditions are such that this dignity is marginalized and/or the burden of caregiving begins to destroy the caregiver, the higher value may be to "honor and respect" by allowing a third party to manage the challenge.

> But when the parent begins to destroy the child even in cases where the parent is not consciously doing so, the child may save himself or herself and observe the command to "honor," that is, care for the parent, by proxy. In such a case, the child "respects" the parent best by warding off the development of such hostility toward the parent that breaches of filial responsibility will become inevitable, destroying both parties' sense of worth, love and dignity.[22]

There is no hard-and-fast guide for this. That is why the case-by-case, or contextual, aspect of Jewish tradition and values is so important. Each case *is* different as each person and family define dignity and sanctity, as well as honor and respect, in their own ways. The wild cards of autonomy, technology, and one's own spirituality also have an impact on all of these caregiving challenges that we continually face. Yet the foundation in Judaism for all of these decisions remains the dignity and sanctity of the human being and the preservation of that human life in dignity and sanctity. Jewish theology sees each of us as created in that divine image and, thus, by the mere fact that we exist, we have been endowed with that sense of self-worth, dignity, and value.

That ethical foundation is present no matter what age we are or in what condition we find ourselves. The relationship between the human being and God, as manifest in the actions of one human being to another, is the theological foundation for the Jewish approach to health and wellness. The application of that approach remains in our hands as to how we choose to live our lives and follow the ethical principles of Jewish tradition. Context and choice remain paramount, as Dr. Ruth Langer explains in her interpretation of Maimonides:

> Turning to a nursing home placement, in home nursing services, or some part-time arrangement that relieves the child of fulltime caregiving is thus fully appropriate under Jewish law when the child's attempts to provide care will result only in a deterioration of the relationship, causing the child to manifest a lack of honor or reverence for the parent. The point at which this occurs will obviously vary from case to case, and each decision must be reached individually.[23]

THE CHALLENGES OF THE AGING BABY BOOM GENERATION

The challenges of medical technology and the questions of how to make informed Jewish choices as life ends are questions that will continue to challenge us. Yet I would suggest that these may not be *the* questions that will provide theologians and scholars with concerns in the coming decades. The revolution in longevity has given rise to what may be the most profound question of our time: What do we do with the time that we have been granted?

The baby boomer generation expects longevity. It is a massive consumer of health-related enterprises from supplements to body part replacements. The boomers are living longer and living, in many cases, better than their parents' generation, the first generation of longevity pioneers. Thus, the real challenge to us in the coming decades will be in how we come to deal with *time*! It is in this context that I return to the text to again focus on Genesis 3 and God's initial question, "Where are you (*Ayecha*)?"

Time has allowed many of us to focus on those "why" questions that underscore the search for meaning and purpose. Why was I born? Why must I die? Why am I here? What is my purpose in life? It is these questions that form the greatest intellectual, spiritual, and academic challenge for us, and their importance is a direct result of the revolution in longevity. It is as if a prophecy of Dr. Viktor Frankl has been realized when he cautioned that the question of what is the meaning of life is not the question of life, rather it must be how we ask "what life expect[s] from us."[24] How can we live so our life has meaning? In doing so, we begin to answer *ayecha*. How do we frame those answers in this age of longevity? We frame our answers through the prism and power of personal relationships.

I believe that the most powerful aspects of our lives, especially as we grow older, are the relationships that we form and attempt to maintain. It is through these relationships that we define our own self and find, in a very real sense, our own answer to the "why" questions of Genesis 3. Those questions, and our search for our answers, become increasingly important because as we age, we gradually confront the reality of our own mortality. This really is the greatest challenge before us. All other issues pale into insignificance. Longevity has given us time and that time has allowed us to confront our own sense of finity. This is why the texts and the fundamental values of Judaism are so important. We are created in relationship (through our parents and with God) and, as a result, are endowed with our own unique sense of self. It is through relationships with people and the world that we come to realize our place in the universe, our own unique answer to God's *ayecha*. We return to the basics in that, as we seek to embrace and celebrate health and wellness, we do so in order to be able to live our lives and seek the answers to those "why" questions. As our own mortality becomes more present, the search, the seeking of meaning, becomes more powerful. Implicit in our search is another text that I suggest is very instructive in understanding one of, if not the, great spiritual challenges that lay before us.

In Genesis 2:18, we are told that it is not good that mankind is alone. The Hebrew word that leaps out is the word *l'vado*, which is translated as "alone." Let me suggest that this verse gives us an insight into what lies ahead. Let me suggest that much of the evolving challenge to our aging population rests upon two words, two concepts, two sides of the same coin. Two Hebrew words form this challenge: *lev* and *l'vado*. The word *lev* means heart and I suggest that it symbolizes the idea of love. Thus, "love" and "alone" form the tension that presents itself as the challenge before us. Why love and alone? Simply put, it is love that remains the primary drive and need of each of us. It is not necessarily romantic love; rather, it is the sense of being needed, of needing love and to love, of being in relationship with other human beings. Why? Because as we grow older and become more aware of our own mortality, we fear being alone. The antidote for that sense of isolation and aloneness is community and relationships. The greatest challenge for us as a society in the emerging longevity era will be to see how we can keep people from being isolated and alone. How we keep people in touch with and involved with other human beings, no matter what their stage of life and condition, will test every aspect of society.

Heschel confronts these significant questions from a context that sees the search for meaning as something greater than just a drive for personal contentment. He raises the level of discussion of what we want for the rest of our lives from the mundane and temporal to the spiritual and transcendent:

What I look for is not how to gain a firm hold on myself and on life, but primarily how to live a life that would deserve an eternal Amen. It is not simply a search for certitude (though that is implied in it) but for personal relevance, for a degree of compatibility; not an anchor of being but a direction of being. It is not enough for me to be able to say "I am"; I want to know *who I am,* and in relation to whom I live. It is not enough for me to ask questions; I want to know how to answer the one question that seems to encompass everything I face: What am I here for?[25]

The gift of time is perhaps the greatest gift of life. We are now standing at the precipice of this revolution in longevity and with it we are seeing attempts to create a revolution in time. Scientists are exploring the "secrets" of aging, from diet to cell structures, in hopes of unlocking more years, perhaps even to Moses' legendary one hundred and twenty. Yet the question will remain, for what? Is it just time we are seeking, or time with a sense of meaning and purpose? Is it time that we will spend alone, or will it allow us to foster relationships, create new avenues for intimacy, and drive back the veil of being *l'vado*, alone?

The challenge before us may be to invest the time we have in seeing that time as an opportunity for fulfillment. Perhaps that is why increasing numbers of baby boomers are redefining "retirement" by saying to themselves that the gift of time is allowing them to do what they have always wished that they could do.

Again, Heschel serves as a contemporary prophet, for he anticipated the love-alone tension implicit in our search for *ayecha* in a speech at the 1961 White House Conference on Aging:

May I suggest that man's potential for change and growth is much greater than we are willing to admit and that old age be regarded not as the age of stagnation but as *the age of opportunities for inner growth*? The old person must not be treated as a patient, nor regard his retirement as a prolonged state of resignation. The years of old age may enable us to attain the high values we failed to sense, the insights we have missed, the wisdom we ignored. They are indeed formative years rich in possibilities to unlearn the follies of a lifetime, to see through inbred self-deceptions, to deepen understanding and compassion, to widen the horizon of honesty, to refine the sense of fairness.[26]

A great challenge for us as we move forward, then, will be in the emerging longevity revolution now being spearheaded by the aging of the baby boom generation. Jewish tradition sees this revolution in the context of our own historical and theological framework. We are in relationship with God and this is the fundamental and primary relationship we have. By the fact that we have been created with that divine spark within us, we are endowed with dignity and value and worth. In living that life, we seek to answer God's initial call from Genesis 3 of "*Ayecha*?" where are you? The search for our answers to that question, and the "why" questions that arise from that first question, form the curriculum of our lives, especially as we age. As we confront our own mortality, we come to realize that the most powerful need we have is to be in relation with other human beings, to love and be loved; and the greatest fear may be the absence of that sense of relationship and thus the fear of being alone in light of the ultimate aloneness that awaits us all. The gift of time is ours to use as we see fit, and the challenge before us will be how we come to use that time and to embrace its meaning for us. To ensure the time is as useful as possible and to ensure that we are able to stand in relationship in life with God, we understand that health and wellness are a primary concern; for our body and life, as gifts, need to be respected and nurtured, for that is one major way in which we honor that fundamental relationship with God.

Life and health, body and spirit are all part of the same creation, and, thus, the Jewish model for health and wellness, no matter what the age we are, is a holistic interconnected model. We are part of a creation, part of a dynamic evolving life, and have been endowed with dignity and worth even up to the last breath of life. In looking ahead, we may look for a way that can structure all of this into a system that we can apply to our own lives. None of this makes sense unless it is applicable to each of us. Again, we return to classic texts and values to provide a formula for how to move forward in this new age of longevity. The formula speaks to four classic values that build on each other and that can be seen as a way to view how we can move forward. These values can give us substance and direction to how we can conceptualize the message of healthy aging within the context of our own relationships and our own struggle for meaning. The values of *b'riut* (health), *r'fuah* (healing), *sh'leimut* (wholeness), and *k'dushah* (holiness) form a foundation for dealing with the challenges of longevity.

We wish to stay healthy and we know that health is a way in which our relationship with God is manifest. We know that health is so critical that texts have been interpreted to allow for the advances in medicine that we enjoy today. Health is a primary value in Jewish tradition. Likewise, healing is health's companion in many instances. We pray for healing and we understand that healing may take place even if a cure cannot. The tradition speaks of healing the body and mind and soul. Healing is an important component in maintaining health and when the two are in harmony, we may reach a state of wholeness. This holistic approach to life is, I feel, part of how Judaism responds to and acknowledges the ideal relationship with God and the ideal relationship we seek with others. We wish to live in harmony—harmony of mind, body, and spirit—not only with others, but with our own self. This is the goal of life, in a way, to live in wholeness, completeness. In doing so, in merging health and healing with wholeness, we reach a state of holiness.[27]

The challenges of the emerging longevity revolution present our society with opportunities to find creative responses in the field of social and economic policy. For people of faith, that revolution is now presenting us with a unique opportunity to re-vision and redefine how we bring a sense of the sacred to this new multigenerational cohort that is now reshaping religious life. Failure to respond in meaningful ways may see religion for this cohort being relegated to the margins of their lives.

NOTES

1. Leviticus *Rabbah* 34:3.
2. *Mishkan T'filah: A Reform Siddur*, ed. Elyse D. Frishman (New York: CCAR Press, 2007), 33.
3. Numbers 12:13 (NJPS).

4. Laura J. Praglin, "Jewish Healing Tradition in Historical Perspective," in *The Mitzvah of Healing: An Anthology of Jewish Texts, Meditations, Essays, Personal Stories, and Rituals*, ed. Hara E. Person (New York: UAHC Press/Women of Reform Judaism, 2003), 5.

5. Ibid.

6. David L. Freeman and Judith Z. Abrams, eds., *Illness and Health in the Jewish Tradition: Writings from the Bible to Today* (Philadelphia: Jewish Publication Society, 1999), xxii, xxvii.

7. Cited in ibid., 134–35.

8. *Yoreh Deah* 336:1, cited in Fred Rosner, *Contemporary Biomedical Issues and Jewish Law* (Jersey City, NJ: Ktav, 2007), 165.

9. Cited in Fred Rosner, *Medicine in the Mishneh Torah of Maimonides* (New York: K'tav, 1984), 63.

10. J. D. Eisenstein, ed., *Ozar Midrashim: A Library of Two Hundred Minor Midrashim* (New York: Bloch, 1915), 2:580–81. A more comprehensive examination of this text can be found in Elliot N. Dorff, *Matters of Life and Death: A Jewish Approach to Modern Medical Ethics* (Philadelphia: Jewish Publication Society, 1998), 333n45.

11. Asaph date is uncertain. Scholars seem to indicate dates between the third and seventh century of the Common Era.

12. Quoted in Freeman and Abrams, *Illness and Health in the Jewish Tradition*, 159–60.

13. Abraham J. Heschel, "The Patient as a Person" [1964], in *The Insecurity of Freedom: Essays on Human Existence* (New York: Farrar, Straus and Giroux, 1966), 24–38, quotation on 33.

14. Andrew Weil, *Spontaneous Healing: How to Discover and Enhance Your Body's Natural Ability to Maintain and Heal Itself* (New York: Knopf, 1995), 122.

15. Mordechai Reich, "Some Insights into Maimonides' Approach to Mental Health Issues," in *Moses Maimonides: Physician, Scientist, and Philosopher*, eds. Fred Rosner and Samuel S. Kottek (Northvale, NJ: Jason Aronson, 1993), 167–72, quotation on 168.

16. "Compassionate and Comfort Care Decisions at the End of Life," Resolution Adopted by the General Assembly of the Union of American Hebrew Congregations, November 30–December 5, 1995, accessed at http://urj.org/life/community/health/bioethics/?syspage=article&item_id=2014.

17. Solomon B. Freehof, "Relieving Pain of a Dying Patient" [1975], in *American Reform Responsa: Collected Responsa of the Central Conference of American Rabbis 1889–1983*, ed. Walter Jacob (New York: CCAR Press, 1983), 253–57.

18. Exodus 20:12 and Deuteronomy 5:16.

19. Leviticus 19:3.

20. Benjamin Freedman, *Duty and Healing: Foundations of a Jewish Bioethic* (New York: Routledge Press, 1999), 124.

21. Michael Chernick, "Who Pays?: The Talmudic Approach to Filial Responsibility," in *That You May Live Long: Caring for Our Aging Parents, Caring for Ourselves*, eds.

Richard F. Address and Hara E. Person (New York: UAHC Press, 2003), 94–102, quotation on 95–96.

22. Ibid., 101.

23. Cited in Richard F. Address, *Seekers of Meaning: Baby Boomers, Judaism and the Pursuit of Healthy Aging* (New York: URJ Press, 2011), 89–90.

24. Viktor E. Frankl, *Man's Search for Meaning* [1959] (New York: Washington Square Press, 1988), 98.

25. Abraham Joshua Heschel, *Who Is Man* (Stanford, CA: Stanford University Press, 1965), 52–53.

26. Abraham Joshua Heschel, "To Grow in Wisdom" [1961], in *Insecurity of Freedom*, 78.

27. For a fuller explanation of this formula, see Address, *Seekers of Meaning*, 113–38.

DAYLE A. FRIEDMAN

3. DWINDLING OR GRATEFUL

Toward a Resilient Old Age

"Marjorie," a retired business owner and community activist, was seventy-seven when we met at a café in her downtown neighborhood to explore whether she would support the work I was doing in aging and Judaism. I was happy she had been able to fit me in amidst her busy schedule of meetings, university classes, classical concerts, and travels. Casually dressed, she was brusque and businesslike, as always. She had previously told me that aging "wasn't her thing." With eyes bright with excitement, she had described her passionate commitment to creative outreach to young Jews. I found her quite intimidating!

This time, though, our conversation took a different turn. Maybe it was because she momentarily lost her footing as she reached for a napkin she had dropped. Or perhaps it was because I asked her a question that evoked a response on a different plane. I had inquired about what kept her so vibrantly engaged at her age.

Marjorie answered, "As I see it, there are only two choices at my stage of life. You can dwindle, as so many people I know do—just get narrower and narrower, 'til all you can talk about is your aches and pains. Or you can be grateful. I prefer the latter. I have so much in my life and I am going to enjoy every concert, every class, every project, and every moment with my kids and grandkids."

How do you end up grateful and not dwindling? According to Marjorie, this existential stance was the fruit of hard work she had done since midlife, facing her "dark side" through therapy and personal growth programs, endeavoring to grow and change so that she could focus on what was truly important now.

Marjorie had a chance to "walk the walk" a year after our chat, when she faced a recurrence of cancer. When the diagnosis was confirmed, she announced to her family and friends that she had no intention of spending her final days or months in the desperate pursuit of treatments unlikely to significantly prolong her life. Instead, she went home on hospice care. She spent time with each of her many grandchildren and gave each an object from her home to remember her. She corresponded by Care Pages with scores of friends from various parts of her life. She entered residential hospice to get help with pain control and continued her visits and correspondence. She died six weeks later, at peace, grateful, and an inspiration to all who knew her.

I have spent the last quarter of a century exploring the terrain of later life. I have met many elders who have dwindled. Faced with inevitable challenge and limits, they are reduced, and often bitter. They are alive, but not necessarily glad that they are. Some of them I met when I was a nursing home chaplain would confide, "I know I shouldn't say this, but I pray every night that I won't wake up." Yet others bubbled with enthusiasm, or passion, or love, like Sophie, a ninety-five-year-old nursing home resident who would read the daily newspaper and weep as she learned of violence among young people in her old neighborhood.

As I reflect on the elders that I have accompanied as a chaplain and rabbi, I am continually awed by the radically varied ways that individuals walk this path and meet the blessings and vicissitudes along the way. How can we understand the awesome and magnificent journey beyond midlife? And what explains how some of us flourish, like Marjorie, and others flounder amidst its challenges?

These questions are critical, as they point to what, if any, role spirituality and religion might have in fostering resiliency. They call on us to think in new ways about how we prepare for the challenges of aging. And they set the agenda for both practical communal endeavor and research.

In this essay, I shall explore a way of thinking about the spiritual journey of growing older. I shall propose Lifespan Judaism, a new approach to aging for the Jewish community, and examine the practical and research implications that flow from it.

LIFE'S FINAL EXAM—A PHENOMENOLOGY OF GROWING OLDER

In order to frame the experience on the path beyond midlife, I suggest we draw on a teaching from the Kabbalah. Rabbi Isaac Luria, the great sixteenth-century mystical sage, taught this: the world we live in, the life we have, is born out of shattering (*shever*). Through a devastating cosmic accident, God's light could not be contained by the "vessels" that God had created to be the world. The vessels shattered.

The light that was abundant and everywhere before creation became hidden and dispersed—encased in shards (*klipot*) of the vessels that were intended to hold it. The divine became limited and concealed in a world of darkness. Our human task is to find and to liberate the dispersed sparks, and thus bring repair (*tikkun*) and redemption to this broken existence. We reclaim the sparks through mitzvot, holy acts of *torah*, *avodah*, and *gemilut hasadim*.

THE APPLICATION TO LATER LIFE: THE MAP

This teaching can be a template for later life. *Shever*-shattering and *tikkun*-redemptive repair are central aspects of the journey beyond midlife.

Shever: Shatterings and Loss

In the journey beyond midlife, shatterings are rampant, inevitable, and recurrent. We will all face them. We will have to face the shattering of losing dear ones. I will never forget when I was forty and a dear friend died suddenly and shockingly at age forty-six. A wise but blunt friend offered me very unwelcome words when she said, "Welcome to middle age." I was outraged, but of course, my friend was right—as we move through and beyond midlife, we eventually lose parents, friends, and, too often, siblings and partners. Some of their deaths will be sudden and tragic, some will be at a ripe age and peaceful, but nonetheless, their absences leave holes in our hearts and our lives.

As we move past midlife, we may also encounter the shattering of changing roles. Most of us will not work forever, and, even if we do, our companies or organizations will not stay the same, so our roles will not remain static. If we have been community volunteers or leaders, we will eventually have to voluntarily or involuntarily move aside for those who are coming up behind us. Those of us who are parents see our kids grow up and have to figure out who we are to them, and who we are in the world, when we are no longer cook, homework coach, driver, playmate, and daily guide. Our parents grow older and become frail. Instead of leaning on them for help and support, we are suddenly called to care for them, to guide them, even when they do not want us to, through complicated and often treacherous choices.

In the second half of life, some of us will contend with the shattering of disillusionment. Perhaps we will be crushed by the gap between our youthful idealism and the tenacity of the world's problems. Perhaps we will be discouraged, or become cynical. Or perhaps we will wonder: Is this all there is? A friend told me about a colleague she met at a professional conference. This tenured professor was grieving the fact that though she had written three books, none had ever been reviewed in the most prestigious journal in her field. She will never fully meet her expectations and dreams. Nor will we.

And, of course, we will encounter the shattering of the fantasy that we will always be well, always be independent, always be. Our bodies will change—at some point or other, we all do a double take when we look in the mirror and see a strange person with unexpected wrinkles or gray hair stare back at us. That is hard, but there will be much harder ahead. Whether it is the subtle loss of name retrieval or the humbling struggle with chronic illness or it is the confrontation with disability and dependency, our habituated ways of being will surely be shattered.

In the wake of shattering, the light that was in our lives has been dispersed, and it is hidden—at the moment of cataclysm, we cannot perceive it. To use the language of Luria, the sparks-*nitzotzot* are encased in shells or shards—*klipot*. When faced with shattering, we feel grief, disgust, fear, anger, abandonment, disappointment, and confusion. Our deepest wish is, "Why can't it stay the way it was?" We want to return to Eden. We say, *hashiveinu*, take us back there, God.

Tikkun: Repair and Redemption in the New Creation

We are wounded by shatterings, and yet we are alive. Our life is thus a new creation—one that emerges out of the shattering. We might wish to go back, but we are not given that choice. The only existential choice is whether we will dwell in the darkness or seek (and lift up) the sparks of light hidden within our new reality. This is what Luria called "*tikkun*—repair."

I have seen many people who cannot get past a shattering, who remain forever immersed in darkness, despair, and bitterness. But I have also seen the ones who reach for the light, such as "Wilma," a beloved member of the nursing home community who lost her speech after a devastating stroke but managed to communicate love, humor, and kindness through persistence, gestures, and sheer force of personality. Wilma was stripped of so many things we count on to make us human: her speech, her ability to eat, her physical attractiveness. Yet in the face of hardships that would prompt most people to withdraw in anger or frustration, Wilma remained distinctly herself. She found ways to draw others to her with love, creativity, and passion. She sought—and found—the holy sparks and illuminated the darkness for all she touched.

The shatterings of aging are life's final exam. We may have decades of good health and opportunity beyond midlife, but we will certainly, at some point, also encounter loss, limits, and mortality. Our contemporary culture endeavors to defeat aging so as to escape these challenges. We are barraged daily with invitations to "defy" aging through hair color, wrinkle treatments, vitamins, or unproven medical treatments. We hide the oldest old away in institutions and senior communities as if, through physical distance, we could protect ourselves from the realities they courageously face. They know, and we will eventually learn, that no amount of ginkgo biloba, or Pilates class, or cosmetic surgery will keep illness, loss, and death at bay.

What I want to know is what equips us for this? What can foster resiliency—the capacity to see the sparks—to tap into gratitude, compassion, and engagement even as we suffer shatterings? What will answer Robert Butler's piercing question: "Why survive?"[1] Through my years as a nursing home chaplain, I have seen how powerfully Jewish practice and community can foster meaning, connection, and inspiration for those who are already old. Now I wonder: What if these Jewish resources could actually help us to get ready for life's "final exam"?

LIFESPAN JUDAISM: A TRANSFORMATIVE APPROACH TO AGING

It seems to me that the difference between what Marjorie called "dwindling" and "grateful" has partly to do with personality and emotional makeup, but also can be affected by preparation. We can face all of these shatterings of later life with maximal resilience if we can tap into virtues, wisdom, and spiritual tools we have acquired along the way. As geriatrician Bill Thomas teaches:

> You are, on this very day, living the life you will remember as an elder.
> You are the living breathing human being upon which your elder self will base all of his or her most important and valuable stories.
> You are, literally, an elder in the making.[2]

I would like to suggest that Judaism can provide a spiritual curriculum to help us to grow and deepen in adulthood. My colleague, Dr. Beulah Trey, and I call this approach Lifespan Judaism.[3] Lifespan Judaism is a way of looking at the content and structure of Jewish life and community and an approach to shaping it as well. In order to outline this approach, we shall first explore notions of spiritual development.

Understanding Adult Spiritual Development

From the time we leave our parents' homes until the moment of our deaths, we have the opportunity to grow and learn. Scholars have attempted to analyze the progression of spiritual development in various ways. Some theorists, such as James Fowler,[4] M. Scott Peck,[5] and Harry Moody,[6] posit that we pass through a linear, predictable progression from our childhood faith and character to a mature spiritual outlook. Others, such as Ruth Ray and Susan McFadden,[7] and Robert Atchley,[8] critique linear stage models as too narrow to capture the complexity and variety of spiritual experience. McFadden and Ray suggest that spiritual capacity and identity are developed within a group or community (the web) and over the course of a lifetime of encounters with others (the quilt). Atchley posits ongoing cycles of spiritual development, in which an emerging interest or question propels the individual toward learning, practice, exploration, and a new sense of integration.

Perhaps most useful to us is the perspective of psychologist Robert Kegan.[9] Kegan teaches that as we face each new stage or task in life, we are "in over our heads." We experience a gap between what we have prepared for and what we are encountering. According to Kegan, it is in that gap that growth and development occur. I would suggest that the content and context of Jewish life can offer precisely the resources to support growth and development as we move through life, a life preserver available when we face the inevitable moments of being in "over our heads," and to foster the accrual of tools and traits to make us resilient in the face of the challenges of aging.

THE SPIRITUAL CURRICULUM OF JEWISH LIFE

Content

Jewish learning, or *torah*, offers wisdom to frame our experiences. The sages say of the sacred text, "Turn it and turn it for all is within it."[10] Through the annual cycle of reading of the Torah (Pentateuch), Jews encounter the same stories and laws every year. In reading and studying the text, we inevitably find that it has relevance for our lives' current dilemmas. In the broader sense, studying Jewish texts written through the ages provides a lens through which to see our own experience, a validation that our questions are not ours alone, and a connection to values, norms, and inspiration.

Jewish spiritual practice (*avodah*—sacred service) provides us with the opportunity to transform time by living in cycles of significant moments. The sacred cycles of the week, month, and year are punctuated by rituals that call our attention—to time itself and to a higher purpose of existence. In the cycle of the week, from *shabbat* to *shabbat*, we learn that work and the mundane tasks of existence are valuable, but that they are only part of our lives. *Shabbat*, the day of rest, enables one to be spiritually refreshed through practice and community.

In the cycle of the year, the holidays and festivals connect us to the entire spectrum of human emotion and experience—from the abject desolation of recalling the destruction of the Temples on Tisha b'Av to the giddy frivolity of Purim; from the solemnity and simplicity of acknowledging sin and praying for forgiveness on Yom Kippur to the exalted joy and gratitude for abundance on Sukkot, the harvest festival.

In encountering these festivals and their themes year after year, a Jew has an opportunity to make meaning and grow deeper. We bring our own current life experience and find resonance, validation, and inspiration. On Shavuot, in reading the book of Ruth, an underemployed young adult might identify with Ruth, who is struggling to find sustenance and relationships, while a newly widowed elder might be intrigued with Naomi, who loses everything dear to her and somehow finds unexpected fortitude and new possibilities.

These rituals help us to hold complexity and contradiction and connect us to community as we contend with being in "over our heads." In addition to the rituals that punctuate Jewish time in the week, month, and year, daily Jewish practices may foster the development and growth of virtues. For example, the Modeh Ani prayer, recited daily upon awakening in the morning, can cultivate a sense of gratitude. Blessings for food, bodily functions, and sensory experiences also prompt consciousness of goodness and fortune that might otherwise be taken for granted. The bedtime recitation of the *Shema* encourages reflection on one's day, as well as seeking and granting forgiveness.

Context: The Multigenerational Community

Not only the content, but the context of Jewish life can foster spiritual development across the life cycle. The multigenerational nature of Jewish community is a rich resource. In an organically integrated community, which synagogues ideally are, those who are further along life's path can be role models and mentors for those who are younger. Those who courageously face illness or disability, or those who rise up from the ashes of loss to reinvent themselves, are guides, even if they are not aware of this. Even more significantly, the teaching and learning, as well as the help and support, can be reciprocal.

Simply by witnessing others traverse life passages, we learn and absorb invaluable guidance. For example, young friends of mine recently married. In their *ketubah*, or marriage contract, which was read at their wedding, they included a startling and moving commitment:

> We will care for each other all the days of our lives. The partner who is blessed with longer life will carry out the last rational request of the dying partner, protecting him or her from indignity and abandonment with tender, faithful presence until the end. The one who lives on will proceed in life with gratitude for the years we shared together and openness to what comes after.[11]

Many tears were shed as Zach and Becca read this promise. Friends of their parents cried as they remembered making wrenching decisions about medical treatment for their own parents. Zach and Becca's friends cried as they faced the intimation that even love as shiny and fresh as these beloveds' would not protect lovers from mortality and suffering. Their grandparents and older relatives wept as they wondered how clearly they had communicated their own wishes regarding end-of-life care and caregiving.

The multigenerational community is an ideal holding environment for the journey of spiritual development across the life span. In being connected to those older and younger than ourselves, we have the opportunity to be learning and teaching, giving and receiving as we are growing and deepening.

IMPLICATIONS OF THE LIFESPAN JUDAISM MODEL

Implications for Practice

Spiritual development is, as we have seen, a lifelong process. If we consciously foster lifelong spiritual development in synagogues and communal organizations, we can contribute to resiliency and well-being for those facing the vicissitudes of later life. Seriously addressing spiritual growth across the life span would require us to rethink the structure and organization of Jewish life. While we have noted that the Jewish community is inherently multigenerational, current institutional structures often mitigate against intergenerational learning and support. Current practice often addresses participants or members in cohort-specific silos—youth are engaged through religious school or youth groups; young adults, if at all, through special outreach efforts; and elders, if at all, through "senior" groups. We are not building a stage-by-stage spiritual process, nor are we fostering maximally nurturing communities.

An alternative vision is the notion of Communities for All Ages. Developed by Nancy Henkin and her colleagues at Temple University's Intergenerational Center, this approach suggests that the most vibrant communities are those that engage and connect members across the life cycle.[12] Leaders who wish to forge communities for all ages need to shape communities that eliminate barriers to accessibility and inclusion and to empower members of various ages to be in interdependent relationships of giving and receiving, teaching and learning.

Creating a Jewish community for all ages is a vital element of realizing the Lifespan Judaism approach. Instead of thinking about discrete programming for each cohort, we can shape programs that are open and welcoming to members across the life span. In order to do this, we must investigate and mitigate potential barriers to participation (timing, cost, physical obstacles, transportation, light, sound). We make sure that the spaces are physically accessible to both strollers and wheelchairs, that lighting is adequate for those with low vision, and that there is transportation for members who do not drive at night. We craft publicity that clearly targets all of the cohorts we want to welcome, so that they know that this program is "for them."

In this Jewish community for all ages, we forge meaningful roles for participants of all ages. We want to ensure that each cohort in our community has opportunities for learning and teaching (*torah*), for spiritual practice and worship (*avodah*), and for giving and receiving care (*gemilut hasadim*). No cohort should be addressed solely on a social level (as senior adult groups and teens too often are). No group should be thought of as simply recipients of care. Each member should be invited and empowered to use his or her gifts (ideas, skills, relationships) to contribute to the community.

We need to create experiences that are relevant to the place in the life journey of cohorts we hope to reach. Just as a classroom teacher employs multiple modalities to address different kinds of learners, so, too, a rabbi, educator, or facilitator can forge a service or program that offers "hooks" to participants in various stages of spiritual development. We can think creatively about the themes of the program or service, and craft multilayered experiences that offer something for many, if not all. For example, Chanukah, a holiday that many Jews associate with children, might be deepened by intergenerational storytelling about themes of freedom and persecution, assimilation, and distinctiveness, as well as through hands-on workshops on cooking, crafts, and music open to participants from all age groups. One could imagine a seventy-five-year-old congregant sharing a memory of struggling with being different at Christmastime with a young adult who is wrestling with what Jewish identity means in her life, or a sixty-five-year-old former Freedom Rider reflecting on fighting for freedom with a teenager wondering how he might change the world. Perhaps members of all ages would sing together in a workshop on songs of freedom, featuring Negro spirituals, Chanukah songs, and South African anthems.

Implications for Research

The Lifespan Judaism approach presents important questions for research, as well as practice. We need to know more about what it is that fosters resiliency among Jewish elders facing illness, loss, or disability. Do we, for example, see differences among those who are involved in Jewish life and those who are not (when controlling for other variables, such as functional capacity or material resources)? Does the length of involvement matter? In other words, are those who have been continually involved in Jewish life across their lifetimes more resilient than those who have been episodically involved?

We would also want to see the impact of the Lifespan Judaism approach on communal life. Would focusing on lifelong spiritual development, and on fostering multigenerational community, result in more vibrant communal or congregational life? Would more empty nesters remain affiliated? Would fostering intergenerational connections have an impact on ageism and attitudes toward elders?

CONCLUSION

Rabbi Sholom Noach Berezovsky, a twentieth-century Hasidic master, taught that each life stage offers a gateway to spiritual connection. We need, he suggests, resources to quell our lowest inclinations and to encourage and support our highest capacities.[13] The Life span Judaism approach to fostering spiritual development across the life span can foster this kind of growth and deepening and can help to prepare us with character and spiritual tools to face the "final exam" of later life's challenges with grace and grit.

NOTES

1. Robert Butler, *Why Survive?: Being Old in America* (Baltimore: Johns Hopkins University Press, 2002).
2. Bill Thomas, "Old Memories, Young Hopes," *ChangingAging Blogstream* (February 23, 2011), accessed at http://changingaging.org/blog/2011/02/23/old-memories-young-hopes/.

3. This material was initially developed in collaboration with Dr. Beulah Trey of Vector Group Consulting (http://www.vectorgroupconsulting.com) for a seminar we taught at the Reconstructionist Rabbinical College in 2010–11.
4. James Fowler, *Stages of Faith: The Psychology of Human Development and the Quest for Meaning* [1981] (New York: HarperOne, 1995).
5. M. Scott Peck, *The Road Less Traveled: A New Psychology of Love, Traditional Values and Spiritual Growth* [1978], 25th anniv. ed. (New York: Touchstone Books, 2003).
6. Harry R. Moody and David Carroll, *The Five Stages of the Soul: Charting the Spiritual Passages That Shape Our Lives* (New York: First Anchor Books, 1997).
7. Ruth E. Ray and Susan H. McFadden, "The Web and the Quilt: Alternatives to the Heroic Journey Toward Spiritual Development," *Journal of Adult Development* 8 (2001): 201–11.
8. Robert C. Atchley, *Spirituality and Aging* (Baltimore: Johns Hopkins University Press, 2009).
9. Robert Kegan, *In Over Our Heads: The Mental Demands of Modern Life* (Cambridge, MA: Harvard University Press, 1994).
10. Translated from Ben Bag Bag in *Pirkei Avot* 5:22.
11. Quoted, with permission, from the *ketubah* of Zachary Teutsch and Rebecca Rosen.
12. Nancy Z. Henkin, April Holmes, Benjamin Walter, Barbara R. Greenberg, and Jan Schwarz, *Communities for All Ages: Planning Across Generations* (Baltimore: Annie E. Casey Foundation, 2005).
13. Commentary on *Parashat Shofetim* in Shalom Noach Barzovsky, *Netivot Shalom al HaTorah* (Jerusalem: Yeshivat Beit Avraham Slonim, 1994).

ELLIOT N. DORFF

4. USING JEWISH LAW TO RESPOND TO CONTEMPORARY ISSUES IN BIOETHICS

INTRODUCTION

First, a matter of terminology. In the early decades of the study of moral issues that arise out of the world of medicine, the discipline that explored those issues was called "medical ethics," and it addressed such topics as abortion and euthanasia, matters that physicians faced in their practice of medicine. Subsequently, however, "bioethics" became the more popular term because it included much more. In addition to how physicians practice their art, "bioethics" also includes attention to relevant social issues such as the distribution of health care and environmental issues such as the treatment of animals in general and in medical research in particular. In recent times it has additionally included attention to how we handle cells, genes, and other body parts of both humans and animals and even plant life.

Although the Jewish sources for making medical and environmental decisions extend as far back as the Bible, Rabbi Immanuel Jakobovits was the first to write a comprehensive treatment of Jewish medical ethics. In a presentation at a conference of the Academic Coalition of Jewish Bioethics that I attended that was, as it happens, a few months before he died, he gave us a retrospective of his work in bioethics. It began when he was serving as the rabbi of a synagogue in Dublin in the 1950s. The large Catholic community there was grappling with questions concerning abortion—which, because of antibiotics and advances in surgical techniques, had just recently become safe for the mother—and end-of-life issues, where antibiotics and other new treatments that could extend life raised new moral questions about how far doctors should go in their efforts to do that, especially in patients suffering much pain. His book *Jewish Medical Ethics*, first published in 1959,[1] shows the influence of that Catholic impetus to examine Jewish sources, for in it he frequently compares Jewish doctrines and practices with Catholic ones.

The same Catholic impetus for Jews to examine their own tradition's views on bioethics occurred in the United States, where Daniel Callahan and his colleagues at the Hastings Center were raising the same issues in the 1950s and 1960s, leading, for example, to Rabbi David M. Feldman's seminal book, *Birth Control in Jewish Law: Marital Relations, Contraception, and Abortion as Set Forth in the Classic Texts of Jewish Law,* published in 1968.[2] The United States Supreme Court's decision in *Roe v. Wade* (1973), which made abortion a constitutional right, and its subsequent decision in *Cruzan* (1990), which established an adult's right to refuse all medical treatment and to require the removal of life support, including artificial nutrition and hydration, provided further impetus for Jews to articulate their own view of these matters, and there has been a plethora of Jewish responses across the ideological spectrum of Jewish commitment in the last four decades of the twentieth century and now in the twenty-first.

Because the Jewish tradition historically has primarily used Jewish law as the medium for making moral decisions, it is not surprising that—ranging from most conservative to most liberal—Orthodox, Conservative, Reconstructionist, and even Reform rabbis have issued legal rulings governing medical decisions. I say "even Reform rabbis" because the Reform movement is ideologically committed to personal autonomy, where each Jew decides what to believe and how to express those beliefs in action, and so the use of law, which announces communal norms, would seem to be out of place in such a setting. Reform rabbis, however, want to root their decisions in the Jewish tradition, and that requires a legal treatment of moral issues, even if, in their view, in the end it is up to each Jew to decide whether or not to follow the guidance of the ruling. In the appendix of this essay, I list a sampling of the books that rabbis of all four movements have produced on bioethical matters together with the websites where readers can access rabbinic rulings of the group, including the most recent ones.

JEWISH METHODS TO CREATE THE MORAL PERSON

It is not only through the medium of Jewish law, though, that Jews have addressed moral matters, including bioethical decisions. Because the Jewish tradition uses law most, though, as its method for making moral decisions, and because I will therefore focus on law in this essay, it is important to recognize at the outset that all of the following factors in the Jewish tradition also play a role—and, indeed, affect how Jewish law is interpreted and applied. In the appendix to my book *Love Your Neighbor and Yourself: A Jewish Approach to Personal Ethics*,[3] I talk more extensively about how each of these factors affects the moral formation of Jews as well as how we make specific moral decisions, but the following brief summary of that material will suffice for our purposes in this essay:

1. *Stories.* The primary story of the Torah is the exodus from Egypt, the revelation at Sinai, and the trek to the Promised Land. As I develop in chapter one of my book *To Do the Right and the Good: A Jewish Approach to Social Ethics*,[4] that story is as central to Judaism's perspective on the nature of the human being and the community and the goal of human existence as the Passion and Resurrection are to Christianity and the Revolution and framing of the Constitution are to the United States. Concrete moral decisions made by members of any of these groups are often rooted in the broad perspectives articulated and taught through these central stories.

Specific stories can also guide our deliberations about new medical procedures. What does the Tower of Babel story[5] tell us about the proper limits of human interventions in the alphabet of the human genome? On the other hand, what does the story of Moses intervening to stop the lashes of an Egyptian taskmaster[6] tell us about our duty to stop pain in our fellow human beings, whether caused by people, germs, or bacteria? Where does our mandate to act as God's agents and partners in preventing and curing disease end and our duty not to play God begin?

2. *History*. No nation that has gone through the exile and persecution endured by Jews can possibly have an idealistic picture of human beings; the evil that people have foisted on each other must be part of the Jewish perception of reality. This is, of course, all the more true after the Holocaust, which, among other things, makes Jews very wary of medical research on human subjects.

3. *Family and Community*. We first learn what is acceptable behavior and what is not from our parents. They thus make us aware of the whole realm of moral norms. They also provide the first motivation to act morally as we try to please them. Thus parents and, after them, siblings and other relatives are critical for the moral development of any human being. Judaism therefore takes care to buttress family life with the commands to honor and respect parents and, conversely, to teach one's children. Beyond these legal boundaries, Jewish family rituals are rich and pervasive, thus strengthening the family further, and this emphasis on the family has been translated into Jewish consciousness through such media as popular literature and even Jewish jokes about family relationships.

As children mature, they come into contact with the larger community. While tightly knit communities can have the negative effects of squelching independent moral analysis and action, such communities can also have morally salutary effects. We learn that we cannot steal Johnnie's marbles on the playground from his and other children's reactions to such behavior. Throughout life, in fact, a strong part of our motivation to follow moral rules stems from our desire to have friends and to be part of a larger community. We also aspire to moral ideals in part because we crave the esteem of other people, especially those near and dear to us.

Family and community also play a major role in health care. Habits of proper hygiene, diet, exercise, and sleep, if fostered by one's family and community, can go a long way toward keeping us healthy. Strong familial and communal ties can convince us that we are responsible not only for our own health care, but for that of our family and community as well. On the other hand, traditional foods or patterns of behavior can make us obese or prone to intoxication or smoking. In sum, just as family and community shape our general moral values and behavior, so they influence our attitudes and actions with regard to health care, both for ourselves and for others.

4. *Leaders and Other Moral Models*. Just as children learn morality first from their parents, so too adults learn to discern what is moral and gain the motivation to work for moral goals from their leaders and from their other moral models. Nobody is perfect, of course, and part of the task in seeking moral leadership is to understand that specific people may be ideal in certain ways and not in others. When some of our political or religious leaders have been shown to have moral faults, that sometimes unfairly and unrealistically undermines our appreciation of their real moral leadership on other matters. Thus the leadership in civil rights shown by Presidents Kennedy and Johnson should not be forgotten just because they were each involved in morally questionable behavior in other aspects of their lives.

Similarly, Judaism uses leaders like the patriarchs and matriarchs, Moses, other biblical people, and rabbinic figures throughout the ages as models of ideal behavior and, importantly, also as models of what happens when you do something morally wrong. In that way, Judaism keeps its leaders from becoming idols while still holding them up as figures to be thought of when deciding on one's own moral course. So, for example, when President Clinton was involved in the Monica Lewinsky affair, many rabbis invoked the David and Bathsheba story to discuss the implications of sexual impropriety on the part of political leaders.

It is not only people with specific offices in society who influence us morally. Teachers, counselors, friends, and even our children and students can show us how to behave. Although Rabbi Judah, the president of the Sanhedrin (or, in another version, Rabbi Hanina), was probably referring to the intellectual knowledge of the Jewish tradition, his famous dictum can equally apply to the moral lessons we learn from it: "Much have I learned from my teachers, more from my peers, but most from my students."[7]

Leaders both reflect and affect our views of bioethics. Consider that many American presidents in the late nineteenth century and the early twentieth century were rotund, precisely at the time when being heavy was considered a sign of health. In contrast, contemporary presidents have either been physically fit or have fought to become so. Beginning with President Eisenhower, the interest of American presidents in fostering healthy habits in Americans generally has also become one of their leadership roles. Other politicians, actors, and models have also clearly played a role in this, sometimes presenting models of health—for women, in particular—who are much too thin.

Many rabbis of the medieval and modern period were also physicians, and for generations Judaism has honored doctors in both clinical medicine and medical research almost as much as rabbis (and now some would say more!). Furthermore, the Jewish community has taken a leading role in encouraging its members to be tested for Tay-Sachs and other genetic diseases before bearing children, and rabbis across the ideological spectrum have ruled that Jews must have their children vaccinated. The Greek model of physical prowess demonstrated in athletic events stood in stark contrast to the rabbinic model of the ideal of the Torah scholar. On the other hand, though, the Torah[8] already asserts that everything on earth belongs to God, including our bodies, and so the fiduciary duty we have to take care of our bodies, which are ultimately God's property, has made Jewish leaders continually concerned about health care. That tenet and a number of other biblical stories and laws have also formed the foundation for Jewish concern with the environment.[9]

5. *General Values, Maxims, and Theories*. The Torah announces some general moral values that should inform all our actions—values like formal and substantive justice, saving lives, caring for the needy,

respect for parents and elders, honesty in business and in personal relations, truth-telling, and education of children and adults. The Torah's laws articulate some of these general moral values, and others found their way into books of moral maxims. The biblical book of Proverbs and the tractate of the Mishnah (c. 200 CE) entitled *Ethics of the Fathers (Pirke Avot)* are two important ancient reservoirs of Jewish moral precepts, and medieval and modern Jewish writers have produced some others as, for example, Moses Hayyim Luzzato's *Paths of the Just (Mesillat Yesharim)*.[10]

So, for example, consider what the following verses from the biblical book of Proverbs might tell us about putting the distribution of health care in the hands of for-profit companies:

> My son, if sinners entice you, do not yield;
> If they say, "Come with us,
> Let us set an ambush to shed blood,
> Let us lie in wait for the innocent (without cause!). . . .
> We shall obtain every precious treasure;
> We shall fill our homes with loot.
> Throw in your lot with us;
> We shall all have a common purse."
> My son, do not set out with them;
> Keep your feet from their path.
> For their feet run to do evil;
> They hurry to shed blood. . . .
> But they lie in ambush for their own blood;
> They lie in wait for their own lives.
> Such is the fate of all who pursue unjust gain;
> It takes the life of its possessor.[11]

Or consider what the following verses from the book of Proverbs tell us about how to respond to medical mistakes:

> My son, if you have stood surety for your fellow,
> Given your hand for another,
> You have been trapped by the words of your mouth,
> Snared by the words of your mouth.

Do this, then, my son, to extricate yourself,
For you have come into the power of your fellow:
Go grovel—and badger your fellow;
Give your eyes no sleep, your pupils no slumber.
Save yourself like a deer out of the hand [of a hunter],
Like a bird out of the hand of a fowler. . . .
Six things the Lord hates;
Seven are an abomination to Him:
A haughty bearing,
A lying tongue,
Hands that shed innocent blood,
A mind that hatches evil plots,
Feet quick to run to do evil,
A false witness testifying lies,
And one who incites brothers to quarrel.[12]

Now obviously how best to distribute health care or to respond to medical mistakes are both issues that are far too complex to resolve on the basis of general proverbs—and hence the need for more subtle tools for making moral decisions, like law—but the directive in the first citation to avoid unjust gain when life is at stake and the guidance in the second quotation to tell the truth and apologize are still good principles with which to approach the complexities these modern issues raise.

Some medieval and modern Jewish thinkers formulated complete theories of morality, depicting a full conception of the good person and the good community, together with justifications for seeing them in that particular way and modes of educating people to follow the right path. Several disparate examples of such theories, each with its own recipe for living a moral life out of the sources of Judaism, include the following: Maimonides' twelfth-century rationalist approach, borrowing heavily from Aristotle, articulated in his code (*Mishneh Torah*[13]) and his philosophical work (*Guide for the Perplexed*[14]); the mystical views of the thirteenth-century Zohar and the sixteenth-century Lurianic *kabbalah*; the behaviorist approach of the nineteenth-century figure

Israel Lipkin Salanter; the neo-Kantian rationalism of Hermann Cohen in the early twentieth century; and the existentialism of Emanuel Levinas in the last half of the twentieth century. Each of these people justified their approach as a Jewish one by invoking Jewish sources to make some of their central claims.

6. *Theology*. As in other Western religions, for Judaism God is central not only to defining the good and the right, but also to creating the moral person. God does that in several ways. First, acting in His judicial and executive functions, God helps to assure that people will do the right thing. God also contributes to the creation of moral character in serving as a model for us. The underlying conviction of the Bible is that God is good, and God's actions are, as such, paradigms for us: "As God clothes the naked, . . . so you should clothe the naked; as God visited the sick, . . . so you should visit the sick; as God comforted those who mourned, . . . so you should comfort those who mourn; as God buries the dead, . . . so you should bury the dead."[15]

Ultimately, though, God serves to shape moral character by entering into a loving relationship with us. That is, the Sinai Covenant is not only a legal document, with provisions for those who abide by it and those who do not; the Covenant announces formal recognition of a *relationship* that has existed for a long while and that is intended to last, much as a covenant of marriage does. Relationships, especially intense ones like marriage, create mutual obligations that are fulfilled by the partners sometimes grudgingly but often lovingly, with no thought of a *quid pro quo* return. For God, as for a human marital partner,[16] we should do what the norms of morality require, and then we should go "beyond the letter of the law" (*lifnim m'shurat ha-din*) to do favors for our beloved. In moral terms, we then become the kind of people who seek to do both the right and the good, not out of hope for reward, but simply because that is the kind of people we are and the kind of relationships we have.

In several places, the Bible asserts that God will punish the Israelites for their sins, and among the punishments listed is illness.[17] Conversely, in many places the Bible asserts that God is our Healer.[18]

Early Christian theologians therefore saw it as illegitimate for human beings to interfere with illness and health, a stance that today is maintained only by Christian Scientists. The rabbis, though, noted that the Torah requires an assailant to provide medical care to cure the victim, thus providing the basis for permitting human beings to engage in health care.[19] They understood the Torah's demand to return lost objects to cover a person's lost health as well, and so medical care is not only permitted, but obligatory.[20] The rabbis interpreted the verse in Leviticus 19:16 demanding that we not stand idly by the blood of our brother to mean that we have a duty to save lives, including, for example, those drowning or accosted by highway robbers,[21] and this duty, they say, supersedes all but three other duties in the Torah.[22] They even went so far as to say that no rabbinic scholar—and, in another version, no Jew—may live in a community without a physician,[23] for that would be endangering each person's body, which belongs to God. Thus Jewish sources have seen doctors as the agents and partners of God in preventing and healing illness, and a Jew must *both* pray to God, the ultimate Healer, for cure *and also* go to the doctor and do what he or she says.

7. *Prayer*. Along with theology comes a life of prayer. Jews are commanded to pray three times each day, with four services on Sabbaths, festivals, and the New Year, and five on the Day of Atonement. Aside from the spiritual nourishment, intellectual stimulation, aesthetic experience, and communal contact that Jewish prayer brings, it also serves several significant moral functions.

One of these is moral education. The rabbis created a framework for daily prayer of three biblical paragraphs constituting the *Shema* and twenty-two one-line blessings surrounding the *Shema* and constituting the *Amidah*, so that Jews would have an easily memorized formula to teach them the essence of Jewish belief. In fact, that outline is as close as Judaism ever got to a creed, an official statement of Jewish beliefs. It announces and rehearses some of Judaism's central values, including knowledge, forgiveness, health, justice, hope, and peace.

Moreover, the fixed liturgy reorients us to think about things from

God's perspective. The vast majority of the fixed liturgy praises and thanks God. This immediately tells Jews that they must get out of their egocentric concerns and think of life from God's vantage point. This alone should help people focus on the important things in life rather than the partial goods to which they may devote too much energy.

Prayer also serves as a way for people to confront what they have done wrong and to muster the courage to go through the process of *teshuvah*, return to the proper path and to the good graces of God and the community. People sometimes are stymied by their sins and by the guilt they feel. Jewish liturgy has Jews asking God to forgive our sins three times each day. Such confessional prayers enable people to relieve the guilt involved in sin so that they can repair whatever harm they have done and take steps to act better in the future.

All of these forms of prayer are important for people's mental health, for they continually reorient worshippers to their central values and perspectives. They also give them an avenue to confront their failings and to resolve to do better, in line with the values announced in the prayers. Whether prayer has a direct effect on health is a matter of dispute, and, as mentioned earlier, the Jewish tradition does not tolerate substituting prayer for going to the physician to learn how to care for one's body and cure it. Jewish tradition does, however, provide ample opportunity to pray to God for healing along with following the doctor's advice.

8. *Study*. While family, community, authority figures, and even God are used by other societies to create moral character, albeit in different ways and degrees than Judaism uses those elements, study is one Jewish method for creating moral people that few other societies use as extensively. Moreover, this is an ancient Jewish method, stemming from the Torah itself. The Torah was not given to a group of elders who alone would know it; rather it was given to the entire people of Israel assembled at Mount Sinai. In keeping with the public nature of revelation in Judaism, God tells Moses a number of times, "Speak to the people Israel and say to them (or command them): . . . ."[24] Moreover, every Jew is responsible to know God's commands and to teach them to their children.[25] To ensure that that would happen, the Torah itself

institutes a public reading of the entire Torah every seven years at which "men, women, and children" were to be present.[26]

By the Second Temple period, the Torah was actually read much more often than that, with small sections read on Saturday afternoons and on the mornings of the market days, Mondays and Thursdays, and larger sections read every Sabbath and festival morning. These selections were arranged so that the entire Torah would be read once every year—or, for some communities, every three years. The reading would commonly include a translation into the vernacular and, on the Sabbath and festivals, a lesson or homily based on the section chanted that day. This helped to ensure that the reading was not merely a mechanical act, but rather a truly educational experience. All of these public readings were part of the regular service, and so Jewish worship is characterized by the combination of prayer and study.

Moreover, the Pharisees made study an end in itself.[27] Thus they say things like this:

> These are the deeds for which there is no prescribed measure: leaving crops at the corner of the field for the poor, . . . doing deeds of lovingkindness, and studying Torah.[28]

> These are the deeds that yield immediate fruit and continue to yield fruit in time to come: honoring parents; doing deeds of lovingkindness; attending the house of study punctually, morning and evening; providing hospitality; visiting the sick; helping the needy bride; attending the dead; probing the meaning of prayer; making peace between one person and another, and between husband and wife. And the study of Torah is the most basic of them all.[29]

As a result, those who teach others have, in the rabbinic view of things, special merit:

> David said: "O Lord, many groups of righteous people shall be admitted into Your presence. Which one of them is most beloved before You?" God answered: "The teachers of the youth, who perform their work in sincerity and with joy, shall sit at My right hand [a paraphrase of Psalm 16:11]."[30]

> He who teaches his neighbor's child is as if he had created him.[31]

The relationship between study and morality goes in both directions: study can refine moral sensitivity and buttress the drive to act morally; conversely, morality is a prerequisite for appropriate teaching and study. Maimonides expresses this latter point explicitly:

> We teach Torah only to a student who is morally fit and pleasant in his ways, or to a student who knows nothing [and therefore may become such a person with learning]. But if the student goes in ways that are not good, we bring him back to the good path and lead him to the right way, and then we check him and [if he has corrected his ways] we bring him in to the school and teach him. The Sages said: Anyone who teaches a student who is not morally fit is as if he is throwing a stone to Mercury [i.e., contributing to idolatry].... Similarly, a teacher who does not live a morally good life, even if he knows a great deal and the entire people need him [to teach what he knows because nobody else can], we do not learn from him until he returns to a morally good way of life.[32]

How, though, does study contribute to morality? It does so in at least four distinct ways:

a. *Content*. The most obvious goal of text study is to inform students about what is right and wrong, good and bad.

b. *Judgment*. In real-life situations, values often clash, and so good judgment in resolving moral conflicts is a necessary asset of a moral person.

c. *Motivation*. Text study can also help to motivate people to act morally.

d. *The moral values attached to study itself*. That is, while study can teach students the content of moral norms and the skills of moral judgment and can even motivate people to act morally, the very act of studying itself can inculcate moral values. Exactly how study accomplishes all four of these goals I discuss at length in the appendix to *Love Your Neighbor and Yourself*;[33] for our purposes here, suffice it to say that study has been used by the Jewish tradition to achieve all four of these goals of moral formation of a person's character.

There is, however, a limit and even a danger to study, and so, contrary to the practice of some ultra-Orthodox Jews today in both North

America and Israel, one is supposed to combine study with gainful employment:

> Rabban Gamliel, son of Rabbi Yehudah Ha-Nassi, taught: The study of Torah is commendable when combined with a gainful occupation, for when a person toils in both, sin is driven out of mind. Study alone without an occupation leads to idleness and ultimately to sin.[34]

9. *Law.* Judaism puts a great deal of emphasis on law as a moral tool—more, I think, than most other traditions, but Islam and Confucianism come close to Judaism in their common emphasis on legal methods to discern moral norms and motivate moral behavior. This is in sharp contrast to classical Christian texts, which have a very negative view of law. The view of the Pharisees as narrow, legalistic, and downright mean people in the New Testament, especially in Matthew, sets the tone for seeing Jews as concerned only with details of rules and not with the broader aims that they have. Paul's description of law as leading people to sin and as the exact opposite of life lived by the Spirit is another major source of Christians' negative views of the law.[35] Society may need laws as long as we live in Augustine's City of Man, but law is not, for Christian writers, the way to know what is right and good. So both the importance of law within Judaism and the disparaging attitude toward it within Christianity motivate me to focus on the role of law in Jewish morality.

Here, again, I discuss the ways Jewish law aids in defining and motivating morality much more extensively in the appendix to *Love Your Neighbor and Yourself*, but a list of how law can and does function morally within Judaism will explain why Jewish writers on bioethics routinely focus on Jewish law in articulating a Jewish approach to modern issues:

a. *Law defines and enforces minimal standards.* The most obvious contribution is simply that Jewish law establishes a minimum standard of practice. This is important from a moral standpoint because many moral values can only be realized through the mutual action of a group of people, and a minimum moral standard that is enforced as law enables the society to secure the cooperation necessary for such moral attainment. Furthermore, there is an objective value to a beneficent act, whether it is done for the right reason or not. Consequently establishing a minimum standard of moral practice through legislation provides for at least some concrete manifestations of conduct in tune with the dictates of morality, even if that conduct is not moral in the full sense of the word for lack of proper intention.

b. *Law helps to actualize moral ideals*. But it is not just on a minimal level that law is important for morality; law is crucial at every level of moral aspiration in order to translate moral values into concrete modes of behavior. A regimen of concrete laws that articulate what we should do in a variety of circumstances can often enable us to act in a morally ideal way when we would not ordinarily do so.

c. *Law provides a forum for weighing conflicting moral values and setting moral priorities*. There are many situations where there is a conflict of moral values and it must be determined which value will take precedence over which, and in what circumstances. Nonlegal moral systems usually offer some mechanism for treating moral conflicts, but they often depend on the sensitivity and analytic ability of an authority figure or each individual. By contrast, the law provides a format for deciding such issues *publicly*, thus assuring that many minds of varying convictions will be brought to bear on the issue. This does not guarantee wisdom, but it does provide a more thorough consideration of the relevant elements and a greater measure of objectivity.

d. *Law gives moral norms a sense of the immediate and the real*. Issues are often joined more clearly in court than they are in moral treatises or announcements of policy because the realities with which the decision deals are dramatically evident in the courtroom and a decision must be reached.

e. *Law gives moral norms a good balance of continuity and flexibility*. Because law operates on the basis of precedent, there is a greater sense of continuity in a moral tradition that is structured legally than in one that is not. On the other hand, through legal techniques like distinguishing cases or, conversely, analogizing them, the law preserves a reasonable amount of flexibility and adaptability. By contrast, moral decisions made on the basis of conscience often have little public effect or staying power; and moral decisions made on the basis of natural law or divine law understood in a fundamentalist way lack sufficient malleability to retain relevance to new situations and to take advantage of new knowledge. A legal tradition, although certainly not without its problems in practice, attains the best balance that human beings can achieve between tradition and change.

f. *Law serves as an educational tool for morality*. Theories of education are obviously many and diverse, but the Jewish tradition has a clear methodology for moral education:

> Rab Judah said in Rab's name: A man should always occupy himself with Torah and good deeds, though it is not for their own sake, for out of (doing good) with an ulterior motive he will come to (do good) for its own sake.[36]

This largely behaviorist approach to moral education is not totally so: as indicated above, study of the tradition is also an integral part of Jewish moral education. But in the end the emphasis is on action:

> An excellent thing is the study of Torah combined with some worldly occupation, for the labor demanded by both of them causes sinful inclinations to be forgotten. All study of the Torah without work must in the end be futile and become the cause of sin.[37]

The same educational theory is applied to moral degeneracy and repentance:

> Once a man has committed a sin and repeated it, it appears to him as if it were permitted.[38]

> Run to fulfill even a minor precept and flee from the slightest transgression; for precept draws precept in its train, and transgression draws transgression.[39]

Thus legally *requiring* people to act in accord with moral rules is a step in teaching them how to do the right thing for the right reason.

g. *Law provides a way to make amends and repair moral damage*. One goal of law is social peace. Legal systems therefore generally provide ways for dealing with antisocial behavior and for adjudicating disputes. A religious legal system like Jewish law also provides a way for overcoming guilt, making amends, and reconciling with God, with the aggrieved parties, and with the community as a whole. That process is *teshuvah*, return, according to which the assailant must do these things: (i) acknowledge that he or she sinned; (ii) experience and express remorse; (iii) apologize to the victim; (iv) compensate the victim in whatever way possible; (v) take steps to ensure that when a similar occasion arises again, the wrongdoer acts differently. In defining that process, Jewish law makes moral repair demanding but possible.

h. *Law helps to preserve the integrity of moral intentions.* We usually construe ourselves as having good intentions, but actions test, clarify, and verify our intentions. Concretizing moral values in the form of law tests the nature and seriousness of our intentions so that we may avoid hypocrisy. It also graphically shows us the effects of our intentions, so that hopefully we will alter those that are knowingly or unknowingly destructive. In other words, law brings our intentions out into the arena of action, where we can see them clearly and work with them if necessary.

APPLYING JEWISH LAW TO MODERN BIOETHICAL ISSUES

When we try to apply Jewish law—or, for that matter, any legal system—to contemporary bioethics, though, we immediately run into the problem that ancient, medieval, and even modern sources did not even contemplate contemporary technology, let alone deal with it. This immediately produces a key methodological issue—namely, how do you gain moral guidance from an ancient tradition for contemporary issues, including those in bioethics?

1. *No Guidance.* One approach is very straightforward: if there is nothing explicitly in the tradition that deals with our situation, we should simply state this and look elsewhere for moral guidance. This approach has several advantages. First of all, it is honest. It does not pretend that the tradition says what it does not say. Second, it takes

seriously the newness of modern circumstances and the need to think thoroughly about how to live nobly in very new contexts; we cannot simply rely on the past to tell us what to do. Third, it is very liberating; it allows Jews to decide the matter for themselves without any limitations imposed by Jewish law. They can then gain guidance, if they want it, from whomever or whatever they wish.

This approach, however, has some serious disadvantages as well. Because modernity has changed our lives not only in bioethical concerns but in virtually every other area of life, the same problem applies to many, many modern issues. If we can apply Judaism to our moral questions only when the tradition has sources that are directly on point, Judaism will not be able to guide us on much of what we need it for most. That will be bad for both Jews and Judaism. Jews will be bereft of any Jewish guidance for important decisions in their lives. Judaism will lose a major source of its attraction and significance for Jews, for even those who are not otherwise religious often look to it for moral instruction, and if they cannot find it, their ties to Judaism will weaken yet further.

That this way of seeing the relationship between Jewish sources and significantly new situations has disadvantages as well as advantages is not, of course, characteristic of this approach alone. Every human theory of anything has strengths and weaknesses, and theories of how law should accommodate new circumstances are no different. Still, the disadvantages of this approach are significant, and so we need to see if alternatives can serve us better.

2. *Everything Is in It*. The opposite end of the spectrum is typified by the rabbinic sage Ben Bag Bag in his comment about the Torah, "Turn it over, and turn it over again, for everything is in it."[40] Ben Bag Bag would clearly not say that about any other text. Thus this approach is built on the theological beliefs that God is the Author of the Torah and that God built into it the answers to all questions that anybody was to ask for all time to come. This is in line with another rabbinic statement: "Even that which a distinguished student was destined to teach in the presence of his teacher was already said to Moses on Sinai."[41]

Clearly it is not the Written Torah itself that contains the answers to everything; it is the Torah *as interpreted anew in succeeding generations* that can produce the answers to all questions. Those who adopt this view believe that when people interpret the Torah, they are not inventing new meanings for it; they are rather *discovering* meanings that God embedded in the text and that we can identify if we only are sufficiently skilled, persistent, and sensitive to see them. Note that classical Jewish texts teach that it is not only the Written Torah that God gave; it is the Oral Torah as well. Therefore one has a much larger corpus of literature from which to draw that enables one to claim that one's rulings have divine authority. One modern who uses this method extensively is Rabbi J. David Bleich, who bases all of his extensive rulings on readings of precedent, whether from the Torah or later rabbinic literature.

The advantages of this methodology are apparent. If you believe that God gave the Written and Oral Torahs and you derive all of your rulings on modern issues from them or the later rabbinic literature based on them, you can claim that your ruling shares in the divine authority of those texts. This methodology also provides a very strong link to the tradition, thus preserving continuity along with authority.

On the other hand, there are significant problems with this methodology. First, the rabbis themselves may have been exaggerating when they said that the answers to all questions for all time are contained in the Written and Oral Torahs. That is, these statements may have been expressions of the love they had for the tradition and the deep meaning they found in it without really intending that everything was to be answered by interpreting it. The tradition, for example, never tells us how to bake a cake or how to fix a broken cart, and I frankly doubt that our ancestors learned those skills by consulting the Torah.

Even if the rabbis of the Mishnah and the Jerusalem and Babylonian Talmuds meant such statements literally, we must recognize that they could state this because the classical Jewish texts that they were creating stretched the Torah to address the issues of their world. Indeed, as Michael Fishbane has demonstrated, the later strains of biblical literature are already interpreting and applying earlier strains, presumably to respond to the needs and customs of their time. There is no guarantee, however, that what they created for their time will fit ours. Indeed, their world changed far slower than ours does, and so the likelihood of their finding answers to their problems in the texts that they inherited is much greater than it is for us.

The most significant problem with this approach, though, is that to gain guidance from ancient texts for modern dilemmas, one often must read such texts out of their own contexts. This distorts their meaning, and that is dishonest. Worse, it applies them to situations that they never contemplated, let alone consciously treated. Thus the results derived from this method may lead to seriously flawed results that fit the modern issue very badly, perhaps even dangerously. One needs to consider the contemporary situation and all its complexities carefully if one has any hope of finding a resolution that is wise and rooted in Jewish perceptions and values. This approach instead looks for any precedent that can be twisted to apply to the current situation and pretends that it gives us the answer to a modern problem, thus wreaking havoc with both the text and the modern issue.

3. *Personal Autonomy.* Is it possible, then, to use the Jewish tradition seriously and honestly to give us moral guidance on issues that it does not treat directly? Modern theorists have suggested several ways to do this.

One approach typical of Reform thinkers, but not exclusive to them, is to highlight the role of the individual in deciding what to do. Reform Rabbis and Professors Jakob Petuchowski, Eugene Borowitz, and David Ellenson, for example, have carefully articulated such an approach.[42] Petuchowski and Borowitz especially emphasize that to be a recognizably Jewish decision, individual Jews must study the Jewish tradition and take into account the import of their decisions for the Jewish community as well as for themselves. Still, in the end, it is the individual who must decide what to do.

Ellenson goes even further in the direction of autonomy: he maintains that asking a rabbi to make a decision based on Jewish law improperly transfers responsibility for the decision to the rabbi and removes it from the person who must decide. Instead of such "*halakhic* formalism," he advocates a methodology in which individual Jews may consult their rabbi and, for that matter, anyone else, but they must assume the responsibility themselves to decide how to resolve moral problems, such as whether and when to remove life support from one's mother, the case that Ellenson uses as his example.

The advantages and disadvantages of this approach are readily apparent. This puts the responsibility of making moral decisions squarely on the shoulders of the individuals who face them. This encourages individuals to take responsibility for their actions. It also prevents them from thinking that they can blame anyone else for what they do, as many of the Nazis did when they claimed that they were simply following orders. Further, it enables individuals to decide issues as they see fit. Aside from the freedom that this brings, it makes it more probable that people will act on what they themselves determine to be moral.

Like its advantages, the problems with this approach are rooted in its individualism. If individuals make their own decisions, in what sense can there ever be a communal norm? Worse, especially because individuals may consult their rabbi and the Jewish tradition as much or as little as they please, what makes the decisions individual Jews make identifiably Jewish?

Petuchowski and Borowitz try to answer this by making the process for making decisions that they map out include knowledge of the Jewish tradition and consideration for the import of individuals' decisions on the Jewish community. Most Jews, however, do not know much about Judaism, especially in problematic moral areas. They also lack the skills of applying the tradition to modern circumstances. Moreover, as Arnold Eisen and Stephen Cohen have demonstrated in their book, *The Jew Within*,[43] modern Jews value personal autonomy much more than their roots in the Jewish tradition, and so the Jewish factors that Rabbis Petuchowski and Borowitz build into their approaches are not likely to be taken seriously enough by most individual Jews to make their decisions recognizably Jewish. This factor is even more problematic in Ellenson's approach, which does not explicitly include these elements.

Another version of this approach has been suggested by Laurie Zoloth-Dorfman.[44] Based on an analysis of the book of Ruth, she suggests that the proper way to make moral decisions is for one person to engage another and respond to that individual's needs personally. Here again the accent is on individual decision making, but it is specifically in the context of a decision involving another person and his or her welfare. This kind of situational ethics is less focused on individuals and their own needs than that of the Reform rabbis mentioned above, and it has the strength of encouraging empathy; but it shares the same problems that the other individualistic theories entail.

4. *Applying Jewish Law Wisely*. I would now like to suggest a methodology for applying Jewish law and the Jewish tradition generally to new moral issues and specifically to issues in bioethics, where so much is new. I have described various aspects of this approach in the appendices of my books on Jewish medical, social, and personal ethics,[45] and I have described its conceptual foundations in my new book on Jewish law, *For Love of God and People: A Philosophy of Jewish Law*.[46] Here I will summarize my own approach a bit more thoroughly than I have described other scholars' theories above and then, as in their case, I will point out its strengths and weaknesses.

I view Jewish law as similar to a human being, with a body and soul. The body of Jewish law, the *corpus juris*, functions in many of the ways that human bodies do, with some parts changing rapidly and others very slowly in order to renew itself and accommodate itself to new environments. The soul of Jewish law, the Covenant, links Jews to God and to each other with the goal of living life in a holy way, a way that takes actions to fix the world and that inculcates in us the desire and character to imitate God and to fulfill God's will for us as we understand it.

The trick, of course, is how to conceive of God's will for us. By and large, we rely on precedent, and Jewish law helps to shape our moral character and achieve our moral goals in the variety of ways that I described briefly above and more extensively elsewhere.[47] Jewish law, however, does not exist in a vacuum: it is like a person's bone structure, which is influenced by every other part of the human being, including its physical, mental, and emotional components as well as its interactions with other people and with its environment. The bones do not change nearly as fast as our skin cells do (we lose and add thousands of skin cells each day), nor even as fast as our bodies replace our blood cells (blood banks will take donations of whole blood from a person only once every fifty-six days); anyone who has broken a bone will remember that it took months to heal. In a similar way, Jewish law remains quite constant relative to other features of Jewish life. Nevertheless, Jewish law is subject to change, mostly slowly but sometimes rather dramatically, just as bones change dramatically in traumatic events like an accident while driving or skiing. In both the slow, evolutionary changes and in the more metamorphic ones, the law must be shaped through continually interacting with Jewish theology and philosophy, historical realities, economic conditions, moral sensitivities, and Jewish goals, just as it has historically been, for it to be both recognizably Jewish and for it to express what the Torah demands, a love of God "with all your heart and with all your soul and with all your might."[48]

In practice, what this means is that on any given moral issue, we must first look for precedents within the corpus of Jewish law. Sometimes the precedent may be directly on point even if the applications of the precedent are quite new. This is the case, for example, with regard to abortion. Now, in contrast to times past, abortions can be done safely, and one might therefore expect that precedents shaped in the past might be appropriately changed now. The metaphysical and legal bases for discussing abortion, however, already exist in the Torah, Mishnah, and Talmud, and they are just as apt within the new medical context as they were in times past. Specifically, based on the Torah and the science of the times, Jewish law asserts that the fetus during its first forty days of gestation is "merely water"; from then until birth it is "like the thigh of its mother"; and it is only when the head emerges from the vaginal canal that it is a full human being.[49] Although we now know that the DNA of the ultimate child is already present in the fertilized zygote, we also know, much more accurately than the rabbis did, that considerable fetal development must take place before one has a full human being. Still, presumably on the basis of miscarriages that they witnessed, they accurately described the stages of pregnancy, for it is precisely around the time that they mentioned that the fetus develops a bone structure and thus looks "like the thigh of its mother." This means that the norms that the rabbis established are still appropriate today—namely, that abortion is usually prohibited, not as an act of murder, which can only happen to a full human being, but as an act of self-injury; that, on the other end of the spectrum, abortion is required when the life or health of the woman is clearly put at risk; and that, when there is an elevated risk to the woman beyond that of normal pregnancy but not so much of a risk that her life is not clearly at stake, she may choose to accept that risk and continue with the pregnancy under careful medical supervision or refuse to accept that risk and abort the fetus.[50] These precedents also form the basis for contemporary Jewish discussions of embryonic stem cell research, where Orthodox, Conservative, and Reform rabbis, speaking for their communities, have all asserted that we should aggressively pursue this promising research, especially on embryos that would otherwise be discarded anyway.[51] Similarly, although the Internet was not available to most people until the 1990s, ample legal precedents in Jewish law exist—together with theological and moral concerns—on which to base a demand that steps be taken to secure privacy on the Internet; the task of modern respondents, then, is to describe what we must do to fulfill Jewish law's concerns in this new arena.[52]

On the other hand, in some areas of the law, such as removal of life-support systems or laws concerning corporations, very little, if anything, exists. Sometimes, in fact, the situation is so different that what does exist clearly does not fit. So, for example, Jewish sources presume that any book that is Torah should be available as readily as possible to the masses, and so its view of intellectual property simply does not apply to anything other than books on Judaism—and even then modern authorities often maintain that authors should have some copyright privileges. How, then, can one formulate an authentically Jewish response to such new issues?

I maintain that one must do what some call "depth theology"—that is, one must identify the foundational concepts and values of Judaism that apply to the area in question and then apply those concepts and values to the case at hand. For that matter, because I believe that Jewish law is part of the living organism that is Judaism, even when legal precedents do seem to apply directly to the case at hand, one cannot simply deduce an answer from those precedents mechanically, as if one were "doing one's sums";[53] one must rather evaluate the precedent in terms of Judaism's long-term commitments embodied in its theology (including its concepts of God and humans), moral literature (the moral norms and goals for life that Jewish sacred literature lays out for us), and customs. Most of the time those factors will reinforce the precedent, but not always. It is for this reason that in all three of my books on ethics, I first delineate the fundamental concepts and values found in Jewish sources on, respectively, issues in medicine, social interactions, and personal matters, for only with these foundational concepts and values in mind can one make authentic and genuinely Jewish moral decisions on concrete issues in that area of life.[54]

Because Judaism, more than any other religion (with the possible exceptions of Islam and Confucianism), tried to formulate its moral inquiries as much as possible in legal terms, most of the time normal legal methods will do just fine in enabling us to use previous legal materials to determine what Judaism would have us do. As I described briefly above and discuss more extensively elsewhere,[55] although the law is not a perfect vehicle to do this, having some distinct disadvantages, it has significant advantages as a tool to probe the depths of moral concerns and produce well-honed directives for our action, advantages that make it superior to the alternatives used by other religious and secular traditions. The law, though, must be used with conscious attention to its foundations in Jewish theology and morality and to its historical context in order to produce wise and appropriate, as well as genuinely Jewish, moral guidance for us now.

Furthermore, individuals, even well-schooled ones, cannot be the sole authorities to do this; rather, the law must be now, as it has always been, the product of the ongoing interaction between rabbis and laypeople acting as a community. Thus, although individual rabbis will and should produce rabbinic rulings ("*responsa*," or *teshuvot* in Hebrew; judicial responses to legal questions), the authority of their rulings rests on their acceptance by both fellow rabbis and the Jewish community as a whole. This is for both practical and theological reasons. Practically, without such acceptance a ruling is simply ignored and, to use a Talmudic expression, simply "flies in the air."[56] Theologically the laypeople have to be trusted as partners with rabbis in discerning God's will for us, for "if the Children of Israel are not prophets, they are children of prophets."[57] Exactly how to balance rabbinic and lay authority is not something that can be easily and universally determined, but what is clear is that law is effective as a moral guide only if such cooperation occurs.

Only if we pay rapt attention to the theological and moral goals set out by the Jewish tradition can we use Jewish law appropriately to give us guidance for our responses to the moral issues of our time. On the other hand, only if we also pay rapt attention to Jewish law and use it to its fullest, invoking not only its content but its methods, can we make decisions on most matters that carry the authority of the tradition and preserve its continuity and wisdom. Both of these processes must be carried out by rabbis and laypeople working in consort, for only then will our efforts to gain moral guidance from the Jewish tradition bear fruit in the way Jews think, feel, and behave. With these methodologies in mind, we can, I trust, make Jewish law for us now what it was for the psalmist:

> The teaching of the Lord is perfect, renewing life;
> the decrees of the Lord are enduring, making the simple wise;
> The precepts of the Lord are just, rejoicing the heart;

the instruction of the Lord is lucid, making the eyes light up.
The fear of the Lord is pure, abiding forever;
the judgments of the Lord are true, righteous altogether,
    more desirable than gold, than much fine gold;
    sweeter than honey, than drippings of the comb.
Your servant pays them heed; in obeying them there is much reward.[58]

APPENDIX: JEWISH WORKS OF BIOETHICS

Some Conservative (Masorti) Authors

Dorff, Elliot. *Matters of Life and Death: A Jewish Approach to Modern Medical Ethics.* Philadelphia: Jewish Publication Society, 1998.

Feldman, David M. *Birth Control in Jewish Law: Marital Relations, Contraception, and Abortion as Set Forth in the Classic Texts of Jewish Law.* New York: New York University Press, 1968. Subsequently published as *Marital Relations, Birth Control, and Abortion in Jewish Law.* New York: Schocken, 1974.

Mackler, Aaron. *Life and Death Responsibilities in Jewish Biomedical Ethics.* New York: Jewish Theological Seminary/Finkelstein Institute, 2000.

Decisions of the Conservative Movement's Committee on Jewish Law and Standards can be found at http://www.rabbinicalassembly.org under the heading "Jewish Law." In addition, the decisions of the Law Committee of the Israeli branch of the Conservative/ Masorti movement can be found at http://www.responsafortoday.com. Conservative/ Masorti *responsa*, both those of the movement-wide Committee on Jewish Law and Standards and those of the Israeli committee, have also been published in book form; see the websites cited above for the names of those books and how to order them.

Some Orthodox Authors

Bleich, J. David. *Bioethical Dilemmas: A Jewish Perspective.* Hoboken, NJ: Ktav, 1998.

Feldman, Emanuel, and Joel B. Wolowelsky, eds. *Jewish Law and the New Reproductive Technologies.* Hoboken, NJ: Ktav, 1997.

Sinclair, Daniel B., ed. *Jewish Biomedical Law*, Jewish Law Association Studies XV. Binghamton, NY: Binghamton University/Global Academic Publishing, 2005.

Spero, Moshe Halevi. *Judaism and Psychology: Halakhic Perspectives.* New York: Ktav and Yeshiva University Press, 1980.

Steinberg, Avraham. *Encyclopedia of Jewish Medical Ethics*. Translated by Fred Rosner. Jerusalem: Feldheim Publishers, 2003.

Legal decisions of the Vaad Halacha (Law Committee) of Modern Orthodox Rabbis (the Rabbinical Council of America) can be found at http://www.rabbis.org. Decisions of ultra-Orthodox rabbis (Agudath Israel) can be found at http://www.jlaw.com.

Some Reconstructionist Authors

Reconstructionist Rabbinical College. *Behoref Hayamim: In the Winter of Life.* Wyncote, PA: Reconstructionist Rabbinical College/Center for Jewish Ethics, 2002.

Teutsch, David A. *Bioethics: Reinvigorating the Practice of Contemporary Jewish Ethics.* Wyncote, PA: Reconstructionist Rabbinical College, 2005.

Teutsch, David A. *A Guide to Jewish Practice: Volume 1: Everyday Living.* Wyncote, PA: Reconstructionist Rabbinical College, 2011. See pages 475–518.

Although the Reconstructionist Movement does not have a formal structure to issue rabbinic rulings for the movement, the Reconstructionist Rabbinical College has a Center for Jewish Ethics (http://www.rrc.edu/ethics-center), which includes attention to medical ethics, and the Reconstructionist Rabbinical Association (http://www.therra.org) formulates resolutions that can relate to medical issues.

Some Reform Authors

Jacob, Walter, and Moshe Zemer, *Aging and the Aged in Jewish Law: Essays and Responsa.* Pittsburgh, PA: Freehof Institute of Progressive Halakhah/Rodef Shalom Press, 1998.

Jacob, Walter, and Moshe Zemer, eds. *Death and Euthanasia in Jewish Law: Essays and Responsa.* Pittsburgh, PA: Freehof Institute of Progressive Halakhah/Rodef Shalom Press, 1995.

Jacob, Walter, and Moshe Zemer, eds. *The Fetus and Fertility in Jewish Law: Essays and Responsa.* Pittsburgh, PA: Freehof Institute of Progressive Halakhah/Rodef Shalom Press, 1995.

Jacob, Walter, and Moshe Zemer, eds. *Sexual Issues in Jewish Law: Essays and Responsa.* Pittsburgh, PA: Freehof Institute of Progressive Halakhah/Rodef Shalom Press, 2006.

Washofsky, Mark. *Jewish Living: A Guide to Contemporary Reform Practice.* New York: UAHC Press, 2000. See especially chapter 6.

Reform *responsa*, including those on bioethics, can be found at the website of the Central Conference of American Rabbis (http://www.ccarnet.org) under the link "Rabbis Speak" and then "Reform Responsa." Reform *responsa* have also been published in book form; see the cited website for a list of such publications.

NOTES

1. Immanuel Jakobovits, *Jewish Medical Ethics* (New York: Bloch Publishing Company, 1959; 2nd ed. with new material, 1975).

2. David M. Feldman, *Birth Control in Jewish Law: Marital Relations, Contraception, and Abortion as Set Forth in the Classic Texts of Jewish Law* (New York: New York University Press, 1968). Subsequently published as *Marital Relations, Birth Control, and Abortion in Jewish Law* (New York: Schocken, 1974).

3. Elliot N. Dorff, *Love Your Neighbor and Yourself: A Jewish Approach to Modern Personal Ethics* (Philadelphia: Jewish Publication Society, 2003), 311–44.

4. Elliot N. Dorff, *To Do the Right and the Good: A Jewish Approach to Modern Social Ethics* (Philadelphia: Jewish Publication Society, 2002), 1–35.

5. Genesis 11:1–9.

6. Exodus 2:11–15.

7. B. *Makkot* 10a, where this is quoted in the name of Rabbi (Judah, the president of the Sanhedrin); B. *Ta'anit* 7a, where it is quoted in the name of Rabbi Hanina.

8. Deuteronomy 10:14.

9. For a good summary of Jewish sources on the environment, see, for example, Arthur Waskow, ed., *Torah of the Earth: Exploring 4,000 Years of Ecology in Jewish Thought* (Woodstock, VT: Jewish Lights, 2000), 2 vols.

10. Moshe Chaim Luzzatto, *The Path of the Just (Mesillat Yesharim)* [1738] (Jerusalem: Feldheim, 2005).

11. Proverbs 1:10–19 (NJPS).

12. Proverbs 6:1–6, 16–19 (NJPS).

13. Moses Maimonides, *Mishneh Torah* [1170–80].

14. Moses Maimonides, *Guide for the Perplexed (Moreh Nevuchim)* [first Hebrew version published in 1190].

15. B. *Sotah* 14a.

16. God is depicted as Israel's marital partner a number of times in the Bible, whether fondly, as in Jeremiah 2:2, or angrily when Israel proves to be an unfaithful lover, as in Hosea 2.

17. Leviticus 26:14–16; Deuteronomy 28:22, 27, 58–61.

18. Exodus 15:26; Deuteronomy 32:39; Isaiah 19:22, 57:18–19; Jeremiah 30:17, 33:6; Hosea 6:1; Psalms 103:2–3; 107:20; Job 5:18.

19. Exodus 21:19; B. *Bava Kamma* 85a.

20. Deuteronomy 22:2; B. *Bava Kamma* 81b.

21. B. *Sanhedrin* 73a.

22. B. *Yoma* 85b; B. *Sanhedrin* 74a.

23. B. *Sanhedrin* 17b.

24. For example, Numbers 15:1–2, 17–18, 37–38; 19:1–2; 28:1–2; 34:1–2; 35:1–2, 9–10.

25. The duty for Jewish adults to learn the Torah themselves: Deuteronomy 5:1. The duty of parents to teach their children: Deuteronomy 6:7; 11:19.

26. Deuteronomy 31:9–13.

27. The Pharisees may have been influenced in this, as Moses Hadas contends, by the Greeks; cf. Moses Hadas, *Hellenistic Culture* (New York: Columbia University Press, 1959), 69–71. I would like to thank Rabbi Neil Gillman for this reference. The rabbis, though, also stressed action, and so their stance toward whether study or action was

more important was deeply ambivalent in a way that the Greek worship of knowledge never was. See B. *Kiddushin* 40b.

28. M. *Pe'ah* 1:1.

29. B. *Shabbat* 127a.

30. *Pesikta (Buber)*, p. 180a.

31. B. *Sanhedrin* 19a.

32. M. T. *Laws of Study* 4:1.

33. Appendix ("The Interaction of Judaism with Morality: Defining, Motivating, and Educating a Moral Person and Society") in Dorff, *Love Your Neighbor and Yourself*, 311–44.

34. M. *Avot (Ethics of the Fathers)* 2:2.

35. On the New Testament's view of the Pharisees, see, for example, Matthew 3:7; 23; Luke 18:9ff, in which they are variously called "hypocrites" and "offspring of vipers." The rabbis themselves recognized the insincere among their numbers, whom they called "sore spots" or "plagues on the Pharisaic party" (M. *Sotah* 3:4; B. *Sotah* 22b). With the exception of the relatively favorable depiction of Rabban Gamliel in the Acts of the Apostles, though, the New Testament paints the Pharisees with quite a broad, negative brush, particularly for being legalistic in their approach to Jewish law—and then, to make matters worse, for hypocritically acting in violation of that law (at least as the New Testament writers see things). For the dispute between Jesus and the Pharisees over the details of Sabbath laws, see Matthew 12:9–14; Mark 3:1–6; Luke 6:6–11; 13:10–17; 14:1–6; John 5:1–18. For Jesus' dispute with the Pharisees over divorce, see Matthew 19:1–14; Mark 10:1–14. For the replacement of law with spirit, see, in particular, Paul's Letter to the Romans 7:1–8:8; 9:30–33, and his Letter to the Galatians 5:16–26.

36. B. *Pesahim* 50b, and in parallel passages elsewhere.

37. M. *Avot (Ethics of the Fathers)* 2:1.

38. B. *Yoma* 86b.

39. M. *Avot* 4:2.

40. M. *Avot* 5:22.

41. J. *Pe'ah* 17a.

42. Jakob J. Petuchowski, "Some Criteria for Modern Jewish Observance," in *Tradition and Contemporary Experience,* Alfred Jospe, ed. (New York: Schocken/B'nai Brith, 1970), 99–128; reprinted in *Contemporary Jewish Theology: A Reader*, eds. Elliot N. Dorff and Louis E. Newman (New York: Oxford University Press, 1999), 292–98. Eugene B. Borowitz, "The Jewish Self," in *Renewing the Covenant* (Philadelphia: Jewish Publication Society, 1991), 284–99; reprinted in Dorff and Newman, *Contemporary Jewish Ethics and Morality*, 106–17. David H. Ellenson, "How to Draw Guidance from a Heritage: Jewish Approaches to Mortal Choices," in *A Time to Be Born and a Time to Die: The Ethics of Choice*, ed. Barry Kogan (New York: Aldine de Gruyter, 1990), 219–32; reprinted in Dorff and Newman, *Contemporary Jewish Ethics and Morality*, 129–39.

43. Stephen M. Cohen and Arnold M. Eisen, *The Jew Within: Self, Family, and Community in America* (Bloomington: Indiana University Press, 2000).

44. Laurie Zoloth-Dorfman, "An Ethics of Encounter: Public Choices and Private Acts," in Dorff and Newman, *Contemporary Jewish Ethics and Morality*, 219–45.

45. Elliot N. Dorff, *Matters of Life and Death: A Jewish Approach to Modern Medical Ethics* (Philadelphia: Jewish Publication Society, 1998); Dorff, *To Do the Right and the Good*; and Dorff, *Love Your Neighbor and Yourself*.

46. Elliot N. Dorff, *For Love of God and People: A Philosophy of Jewish Law* (Philadelphia: Jewish Publication Society, 2007).

47. Dorff, *To Do the Right and the Good*, appendix B, 262–82; Dorff, *Love Your Neighbor and Yourself*, appendix, 311–44.

48. Deuteronomy 6:5 (NJPS).

49. The primary precedents with regard to abortion are Exodus 21:22–25; M. *Ohalot* 7:6; M. *Niddah* 3:5; B. *Yevamot* 69b ("merely water" during the first forty days); B. *Niddah* 17a (distinguishes the first trimester from the rest of gestation); and B. *Hullin* 58a ("like the thigh of its mother" from forty days or the second trimester until birth), with other mentions of this precedent elsewhere in the Talmud. For a thorough discussion of this entire topic, see David M. Feldman, *Birth Control in Jewish Law* (New York: New York University Press, 1968), entitled *Marital Relations, Birth Control, and Abortion* in subsequent editions. For a short summary of this material, see Dorff, *Matters of Life and Death*, 128–33.

50. For a summary statement of the Conservative Movement's Committee on Jewish Law and Standards, see Ben Zion Bokser and Kassel Abelson, "A Statement on the Permissibility of Abortion," in *Responsa 1980–1990 of the Committee on Jewish Law and Standards of the Conservative Movement*, ed. David J. Fine (New York: Rabbinical Assembly, 2005), 817; available online at http://www.rabbinicalassembly.org under the section "Jewish Law."

51. Moshe David Tendler [Orthodox], "Stem Cell Research and Therapy: A Judeo-Biblical Perspective," in *Ethical Issues in Human Stem Cell Research*, vol. 3, *Religious Perspectives* (Rockville, MD: National Bioethics Advisory Commission, 2000), H-4. See also the "Statement on Stem Cell Research" of the Rabbinical Council of America [Orthodox], 2001 and reissued 2004, accessed at http://www.rabbis.org/news/article.cfm?id=100553; Elliot N. Dorff [Conservative], "Stem Cell Research," *Conservative Judaism* 55, no. 3 (Spring 2003): 3–29; accessed at http://www.rabbinicalassembly.org under the link "Jewish Law" and then "Committee on Jewish Law and Standards"; Mark Washofsky [Reform], "Human Stem Cell Research," 5761.7, accessed at http://www.ccarnet.org/responsa/nyp-no-5761-7/.

52. See Elliot N. Dorff and Elie Kaplan Spitz, "Privacy on the Internet," accessed at http://www.rabbinicalassembly.org under the link "Jewish Law" and then "Committee on Jewish Law and Standards."

53. Oliver Wendell Holmes uses this phrase to describe lawyers and judges who mistakenly think that the law can be determined deductively without regard to the values

and concepts that the lawyer or judge has; see Oliver Wendell Holmes, "The Path of the Law," *Harvard Law Review* 10 (1897): 457–78.

54. See chapter two ("Fundamental Beliefs Underlying Jewish Medical Ethics") in Dorff, *Matters of Life and Death*, 14–33; chapter one ("Fundamental Beliefs That Guide Jewish Social Ethics") in Dorff, *To Do the Right and the Good*, 1–35; and chapter one ("Judaism and Ethics") in Dorff, *Love Your Neighbor and Yourself*, 1–32.

55. Dorff, *To Do the Right and the Good*, 270–82.

56. B. *Shavu'ot* 29a; J. *Nedarim* 9a; J. *Shavu'ot* 17a; Exodus *Rabbah* 21:5; Numbers *Rabbah* 12:3; Deuteronomy *Rabbah* 1:22.

57. B. *Pesahim* 66a, 66b.

58. Psalms 19:8–12 (NJPS).

SIMKHA Y. WEINTRAUB

5. GIVE ME YOUR HAND

Exploring Judaism's Approach to the Relationship of Spirit and Health

If a physician cannot give a patient medicine for the body,
he should somehow find and give medicine for the patient's soul.[1]

HEALING AND TORAH: MEANING AND METHODOLOGY

"All beginnings are difficult," we learn in the Tosafot,[2] and, indeed, the task at hand is such a formidable, intimidating one, that one wonders where to start! I am fortunate that inherent in Judaism is always a turning-to-text, a reliance on Torah not only for substance, for the meat of teachings, but for *structure*—for a method of approaching questions and tackling issues. As we shall soon see, Torah is central to healing in Jewish tradition, and so—in beginning to explore the relationship of health and spirituality, or the nexus of Body and Spirit, or the association of religious practice and physiological outcome—the best "launching pad" is to explore the powerful words in Genesis[3] that express the foundational idea that *human beings are created in the image of God.* Let us begin with one expansion of this theme, from the Mishnah:

Human was created as a single individual to teach you that anyone who destroys a single soul is as though he destroyed an entire world, and anyone who preserves a single soul is as though he preserved an entire world; and to preserve peace/harmony among creatures, so that one person not say to the next, "my father is greater than your father," or as some might say, "there are multiple powers in heaven." And to show the greatness of the Holy Blessed One, for while a person stamps many coins from a single mold, and all that are produced come out alike, the King of Kings, the Holy Blessed One, has stamped every person with the mold of the first Adam, yet not one of them is like his fellow. And so, each and every individual is obligated to say, "For my sake was the world created. . . ."[4]

Nice! We draw out of this that every human life is an entire world, that there exists an essential democracy and equality among people, and that each human being, while derived from a single mold, is intended to shine, and to be treasured, in their unique, special differences. The crowning touch is the glorious affirmation that each of us is obligated (not just permitted!) to say: "For my sake was the world created!"

HOW DOES THE "DIVINE IMAGE" MATTER?

But what is the real meaning and import of this "Divine Image"—surely it is not, from a Jewish standpoint, about God's physical appearance. A few other brief quotes from a library of thousands over the centuries will help us:

Man is the axis of the world and its foundation. . . . Though his body be small, his soul is larger than heaven and earth, for through it he reaches even what is above them and the cause of them, the Creator Himself.[5]

Because of the divine image . . . man is superior even to angels.[6]

The one symbol of God is *man, every man*. God Himself created man in His image, or, to use the biblical terms, in His *tselem* [image] and *demut* [likeness]. . . . Human life is holy, holier even than the Scrolls of the Torah.[7]

People often perceive themselves in terms of their constraints as mortal beings. Yet there are times that call for transcendent actions. One must at times do more than one can possibly do, for each mortal is endowed with a G-dly soul and the power to transcend mortal constraints.[8]

Said the Koretzer:

The explanation of the verse, "Let me see your countenance, let me hear your voice" (Song of Songs 2:14) is as follows: God declares to the good person: "Let Me be seen through your face," for God's image is in the countenance of the good person. "Let Me be heard through your voice," for one who hears the words of good people is moved to improve himself.[9]

So our carrying or reflecting the Divine Image means a lot—it suggests our pivotal place on the planet, our sacredness, an intensity of connection with God, and the possibility of at least sometimes transcending our limitations. And what our faces reflect, and our words echo, can actually manifest the Divine. That is quite a lot right there.

BODY AND SPIRIT AS PARTNERS

Since you and I live, very much, in our bodies, and, as we shall see shortly, Judaism upholds an interdependence of Body and Spirit, we must explore that nexus a bit more before moving on:

To whom did David refer in the five verses beginning with "Bless the Lord, O my soul" (Psalm 104)? He was alluding only to the Holy Blessed One, and to the soul. Just as the Holy Blessed One fills the whole world, so the soul fills the body. Just as the Holy Blessed One sees but is not seen, so the soul sees but is not itself seen. Just as the Holy Blessed One feeds the whole world, so the soul feeds the whole body. Just as the Holy Blessed One is pure, so the soul is pure. Just as the Holy Blessed One abides in the innermost precincts, so the soul abides in the innermost precincts. Let that which has these five qualities come and praise Him who has these five qualities.[10]

So our souls are much more than we might think. In relation to our bodies, they are, analogically, what God is to the world. And, in the Jewish understanding, Body and Soul are deeply intertwined:

Everything which came into being was alternately formed of heaven and earth.
When the time came to create human,
there was a tie between the terrestrial and the celestial creatures.
God therefore made human's soul of heaven and his body of earth.
In so doing, God established the harmony of the universe.[11]

Antoninus said to Rabbi: "The body and the soul can both free themselves from judgment! The body can plead: 'The soul has sinned, [the proof being] that from the day it left me I lie like a dumb stone in the grave [totally powerless].' While the soul can say: 'The body has sinned, [the proof being] that from the day I departed from it I fly about in the air like a bird [and commit no sin].'"

Rabbi replied, "I will tell you a parable. To what may this be compared? To a human king who owned a beautiful orchard which contained splendid figs. Now, he appointed two watchmen therein, one lame and the other blind. [One day] the lame man said to the blind, 'I see beautiful figs in the orchard. Come and take me upon your shoulder, so that we may procure and eat them.' So the lame bestrode the blind, procured and ate them. Sometime after, the owner of the orchard came and inquired of them, 'Where are those beautiful figs?' The lame man replied, 'Have I then feet to walk with!?' The blind man replied, 'Have I then eyes to see with!?' What did he do? He placed the lame upon the blind and judged them together. So will the Holy Blessed One, bring the soul, [re]place it in the body, and judge them together, as it is written, 'He shall call to the heavens from above, and to the earth, that He may judge His people' (Psalm 50:4). He shall call to the heavens from above—this refers to the soul; and to the earth, that he may judge his people—to the body."[12]

In sum, Body and Soul are part of an integrated, balanced whole—and are intended to be coordinated in their "program," to function interactively, interdependently, inter-responsibly.

With this background and underpinning, we can appreciate the *Mi Sheberakh LaHolim*, the Prayer for Those Who Are Sick, that Jews offer, traditionally, when the Torah is read in community:

***Mi Sheberakh:* "May the One Who Blessed . . ."**

May the One who blessed our ancestors—
Patriarchs Abraham, Isaac, and Jacob,
Matriarchs Sarah, Rebecca, Rachel, and Leah—
bless and heal the one who is ill:
________ son/daughter of ________.

May the Holy Blessed One
overflow with compassion upon him/her,
to restore him/her,

to heal him/her,
to strengthen him/her,
to enliven him/her.

The One will send him/her, speedily,
a complete healing—
healing of the soul and healing of the body—
along with all the ill,
among the people of Israel and all humankind,
soon,
speedily,
without delay,
and let us all say: Amen![13]

Reflecting a holistic view of humankind, the *Mi Sheberakh* prays for physical cure as well as spiritual healing, asking for blessing, compassion, restoration, and strength, within the community of others facing illness as well as among all Jews, all human beings.

CARING FOR THE BODY

We shall return to the subject of prayer and healing, but, before that, it is important to assert that we don't "just" pray when it comes to health. Because the Body is the container and partner of the Soul, Jews see a binding religious obligation—a *mitzvah*, "commandment"—to take care of our bodies; witness this anecdote about Hillel the Elder, one of the greatest Torah scholars ever, in the first century BCE:

It is written in Scripture: The pious one does good to his/her own soul (Proverbs 11:17). This applies to Hillel the Elder who once, when he concluded his studies with his disciples, walked along with them. His disciples asked him: "Master, where are you headed?" He answered them: "To perform a religious duty." "What," they asked, "is this religious duty?" He said to them: "To wash in the bathhouse." Said they: "Is this a religious duty?" "Yes," he replied; "if the statues of kings, which are erected in theatres and circuses, are scoured and washed by the man who is appointed to look after them, and he thereby obtains his income through them—and is even raised up to be regarded as among the great ones of the kingdom—how much more is it obligatory on me to polish and wash my body, since I have been created in the Divine Image and Likeness; as it is written, For in the image of God God made the human" (Genesis 9:6)?[14]

Indeed, one can perceive a "wellness" or "health-preservation" perspective here—but one motivated not only by personal, selfish objectives but overarching spiritual or religious concerns.

As the first-century philosopher Philo Judaeus expressed, "The body is the soul's house. Shouldn't we therefore take care of our house so that it doesn't fall into ruin?"[15]

And as Rabbi Samson Raphael Hirsch, the great nineteenth-century leader of Orthodox Judaism, summarized: "Respect your own body as the receptacle, messenger and instrument of the spirit."[16]

THE DIVINE IMAGE AND THE JEWS' COVENANTAL RELATIONSHIP

The Divine Image, of course, applies to all human beings, of all religions, races, creeds, nations, centuries, etc. For Jews, the obligations to oneself and to others, and to the world around us, stem from the additional dimension of *B'rit*—the covenantal relationship that we see as represented by the Torah and our unfolding tradition. This two-directional commitment has been understood as enduring and timeless since biblical times:

The Lord God made a Covenant with us in Horeb.... not with our fathers alone, but with us, we who are here and alive this day....[17]

The souls of all future generations also took part when the Covenant was concluded between God and Israel....[18]

One way of describing the Covenant is in terms of our obligation (and privilege) of *imitatio Dei*, imitating the Divine. Note how acts of *hessed*/lovingkindness, including ministering to those who are ill, form the program for such emulation:

R. Hama son of R. Hanina further said: "What does the text (Deut. 13:5) 'You shall walk after the Lord your God' mean? Is it really possible for a human being to walk after the *Shekhinah* (God's Presence)—has it not also been said

(Deut. 4:24), 'For the Lord your God is a devouring fire!' The meaning is: *Walk after the attributes of the Holy Blessed One*. As God clothes the naked—for it is written (Genesis 3:21), 'And the Lord God made for Adam and for his wife coats of skin and clothed them'—so should you also clothe the naked. As the Holy Blessed One visits the sick—for it is written (Genesis 18:1), 'And the Lord appeared unto him by the oaks of Mamre'—so should you also visit the sick.

"The Holy Blessed One comforts mourners—for it is written (Genesis 25:11), 'And it came to pass after the death of Abraham, that God blessed Isaac his son'—so should you also comfort mourners. The Holy Blessed One buries the dead—for it is written (Deut. 34:6) 'And he buried him in the valley'—so should you also bury the dead."[19]

Maimonides—the twelfth-century physician, philosopher, rabbi, and Jewish legal codifier—drove home how essential the maintenance of bodily health was to the Covenant:

> Since by keeping the body in health and vigor one walks in the ways of God—it being impossible in sickness to have any understanding or knowledge of the Creator—it is a man's duty to avoid whatever is injurious to the body, and cultivate habits conducive to health and vigor.[20]

And we hear echoes of this through the centuries; here are two from the fifteenth century:

> When you build a new house, construct a parapet for your roof so that you do not bring blood upon your house, should any person fall from there... (Deuteronomy 22:8). From this we learn that man must not rely on miracles or Providence alone, but must himself do whatever he can to maintain life and health.[21]

> Clothing, bed, table, especially dishes, indeed everything that we ever take in our hands, must be clean, sweet, pure; and above and beyond all, the body, made in the Image of God.[22]

Or finally, a summary from the progenitor of Hasidism in the eighteenth century:

> You may be free from sin, but if your body is not strong, your soul will be too weak to serve God aright. Maintain your health and preserve your strength.[23]

SO WHAT IS "HEALING"? HOW DOES A HEALER HEAL?

What does all this mean for the project of healing? What is the role of healer in a classical Jewish sense? This could be the subject of an entire tome, but, for now, we will visit and summarize just a few central texts from the Talmud. We begin with three powerful stories about Rabbi Johanan, a third-century Palestinian scholar who was also a major healing figure:

R. Hiyya b. Abba fell ill and R. Johanan went in to visit him. He (R. Johanan) said to him: "Are your sufferings welcome/beloved to you?" He replied: "Neither they nor their reward." He said to him: "Give me your hand." He gave him his hand and he (R. Johanan) raised (healed) him.

R. Johanan once fell ill and R. Hanina went in to visit him. He (R. Hanina) said to him: "Are your sufferings welcome/beloved to you?" He replied: "Neither they nor their reward." He said to him: "Give me your hand." He gave him his hand and he raised him. *Why could not R. Johanan raise himself?* They replied: "The prisoner cannot free himself from jail."

R. Eleazar fell ill and R. Johanan went in to visit him. He (R. Johanan) noticed that he was lying in a dark room, and he (R. Johanan) bared his arm and light radiated from it. Thereupon he noticed that R. Eleazar was weeping, and he said to him: "Why do you weep? *Is it because you did not study enough Torah?* Surely we learnt: The one who sacrifices much and the one who sacrifices little have the same merit, provided that the heart is directed to heaven. *Is it perhaps lack of sustenance?* Not everybody has the privilege to enjoy two tables. *Is it perhaps because of the lack of children?* This is the bone of my tenth son!"—He replied to him: "I am weeping on account of this beauty that is going to rot in the earth." He said to him: "On that account you surely have a reason to weep," and they both wept. In the meanwhile he said to him: "Are your sufferings welcome/beloved to you?"—He replied: "Neither they nor their reward." He said to him: "Give me your hand," and he gave him his hand and he raised him. . . ."[24]

Though there is a great deal to derive from these three brief narratives, and some groups (including medical and nursing professionals) have discussed and interpreted them for many hours, let us summarize just a bit of what might be gleaned from this rich text.

In the first paragraph, Rabbi Johanan, laudably, zooms in to visit an ill colleague, and asks him a question, one that seems to be about meaning, coping, or spirit. The one who is suffering responds with an honest reply, rejecting a pious stance that suffering can easily be accepted or understood. At that point, Rabbi Johanan offers the possibility of connecting, of holding hands, and it is through touch and relationship—metaverbal, postverbal connection—that some kind of healing takes place.

Note that in the second story, the healer himself falls ill—"a wounded healer"—and so the distinction, certainly the dichotomy, of healer/healee begins to melt away. Resuming the narrative structure of the previous paragraph, with Rabbi Johanan now as the visitee, the Talmud asks a question that we need to revisit periodically: *Why couldn't the great healer heal him/herself?* The answer points to *a*, maybe *the*, major point in the Jewish approach to healing, and that is: "The prisoner cannot free him/herself from jail"—as community, connection, relationship is of the essence. It is not a matter of this or that practice, but sensing the divine care and compassion through the Divine Image, through fellow human beings, that brings healing if not cure.[25]

Before continuing with the third paragraph, it is important to note one biographical fact: R. Johanan, the healing rabbi, is said to have buried ten children, an unusual degree of infant or child mortality, even for Palestine/Israel of two thousand years ago. To my understanding, in the third paragraph, the weeping initially caused R. Johanan to want to "fix things": he asks (and responds to his own questions) about three concerns that, in classical Judaism, were the subjects of personal prayer, that he imagines his ill colleague is concerned about: Torah, livelihood, and children. When he asks about the latter, about children, R. Johanan returns to his own inner reality, his own personal narrative, his own struggles and resources, and the visitee responds with profound honesty, directness, and power, saying, in effect: "I am weeping because we are all mortal, even someone as beautiful as you." This is a "dust-to-dust" statement, an intimate assertion of our ultimate reality, which brings them very, very close to each other. The two men are able to weep together, joining on a deeply human level, and deeply present for each other.

My teacher and colleague, R. Tsvi Blanchard, in analyzing Maimonides' treatment of the laws of *bikkur cholim* ("visiting the sick"),[26] taught that the essence of reaching out to those who suffer is "shared vulnerability"—the mutual connection of visitor and visitee, not necessarily in having the same troubles, the same diagnoses, or the exact same experiences—but rather a common link of mortality, of exposure, of need, and of concern, love, and support. The theme of mutual weeping of "healer" and "healee" is the theme of a number of stories about rabbis across the centuries.

Over the millennia, Judaism explored and codified when to visit, where to sit, how to be of help and how to avoid being of harm, etc.—in order to maximize the healing quotient, the healing potential, of the interaction and exchange. But that is beyond the scope of this chapter!

Torah and Healing

Another third-century colleague of Rabbi Johanan, Rabbi Joshua ben Levi, illustrates another critical axis of healing, which is Torah. On one truly fascinating page of Talmud, a horrible illness known as *ra'atan* is described in graphic detail, as is their existing manner of treatment, which sounds even more horrifying, even devastating. After this, the Talmud offers:

> R. Johanan announced: "Beware of the flies of one afflicted with *Ra'atan*." R. Zera never sat [with such a sufferer] in the same draught. R. Eleazar never entered his tent. R. Ammi and R. Assi never ate any of the eggs coming from the alley in which he lived. R. Joshua b. Levi, however, attached himself to these [sufferers] and studied the Torah; for he said, "'Let her be like a loving hind and a graceful doe' (Proverbs 5:19); if [the Torah] bestows grace upon those who study it, would it not also protect them?"[27]

What follows in the Talmud is a narrative about God's unusual reward of Rabbi Joshua ben Levi, who overcame the isolation and stigma of *ra'atan* and did what rabbis do—*Torah*—and was granted the opportunity to see his place in Paradise. Stunningly, en route, Rabbi Joshua attempted and almost succeeded in depriving the Angel of Death of his knife, symbolizing terminal illness/death!

We see from this remarkable story that engaging with Torah—and not just with the left brain, not only as a cognitive enterprise but in order to discern God's voice and divine direction, to live in community, to relate to generations past and those to come—is an essential aspect of healing. Not surprising, as Jews and Judaism view Torah as life itself; to quote Hillel again: "The more Torah, the more life."[28]

Torah Heals

Not surprisingly, the same Rabbi Joshua ben Levi is credited as having taught about the healing power of Torah:

> R. Joshua b. Levi stated: If a man is on a journey and has no company let him occupy himself with the study of the Torah, since it is said in Scripture: "For they shall be a chaplet of grace. . . " (Proverbs 1:9). If he feels pains in his head, let him engage in the study of the Torah, since it is said: "For they shall be a chaplet of grace unto your head. . . " (*Ibid.*). If he feels pains in his throat, let him engage in the study of the Torah, since it is said: ". . . and chains about your neck" (*Ibid.*). If he feels pains in his bowels, let him engage in the study of the Torah, since it is said: "It shall be a healing to your navel. . ." (Proverbs 3:8). If he feels pain in his bones, let him engage in the study of the Torah, since it is said: ". . . and marrow to your bones. . ." (*Ibid.*). If he feels pain in all his body, let him engage in the study of the Torah, since it is said: ". . . and healing to all his flesh" (Proverbs 4:22).
>
> R. Judah son of R. Hiyya remarked: Come and see how the measure/dispensation of mortals is not like that of the Holy Blessed One. In the dispensation of mortals, when a man administers a drug to a fellow, it may be beneficial to one limb but injurious to another; but with the Holy Blessed One, it is not so. He gave a Torah to Israel and it is a drug of life for all his body, as it is said: ". . . and healing to all his flesh" (*Ibid.*).[29]

. . . that last quote giving this volume its title!

Later I shall propose a research focus concerning Torah and healing, but for now, let us just establish that the Jewish tradition identifies Torah as a, if not the, major healing resource, for Body and Spirit.

The Healer as "Surety"

Rabbi Johanan, in the third paragraph of the story above, showed how the healer can help through relatedness and mutuality. Jewish tradition is rich in the use of, and reliance on, metaphor, and in exploring the place and program of the healer, this is no less the case. Here is one compelling example in which Rabbi Johanan, again, is the "healee":

> R. Johanan had the misfortune (lit., "was chastised," from heaven) to suffer from gallstones for three and a half years. Once, R. Hanina went to visit him. He said to him: "How do you feel?" He replied: "My sufferings are worse than I can bear!" He said to him: "Don't speak so, but say 'The faithful God.'" When the pain was very great he used to say "Faithful God," and when the pain was greater than he could bear, R. Hanina used to go to him and utter an incantation which gave him relief. Subsequently R. Hanina fell ill, and R. Johanan went to see him. He said to him, "How do you feel?" He replied: "How grievous are my sufferings!" He said to him: "But surely the reward for them is also great!" He replied: "I want neither them nor their reward." He said to him: "Why do you not utter that incantation which you pronounced over me and which gave me relief?" He replied: "When I was out of trouble I could be a surety for others, but now that I am myself in trouble do I not require another to be a surety for me?"[30]

Rabbi Hanina, who, like Rabbi Johanan, was known for his healing skill, establishes that the required relationship of the healer to the one he seeks to benefit is that of a "surety," in Hebrew, *eiravon*, a pledge or a deposit. Incantations, and prayers for that matter, may or may not be effective in achieving desired outcomes, but what is essential is the profound connection of one soul to another, ideally, a linkage so powerful that one "stands in" or "stands up" for the other.[31]

Prayer and Healing

Rabbi Hanina's incantation returns us to the important subject of prayer and healing. Empirically speaking, prayer does not seem to "work" a lot of the time; it does not seem to yield the desired outcomes. Jewish tradition struggled over the centuries to arrive at an honest and evidence-based, and yet also inspiring and encouraging, understanding of *if and how prayer relates to healing*. Consider this discussion:

R. Meir used to say: Two men take to their bed suffering equally from the same disease, or two men are before a criminal court to be judged for the same offense; yet one gets up and the other does not get up, one escapes death and the other does not escape death. Why does one get up and the other not? Because one prayed and was answered, and the other prayed and was not answered. Why was one answered and the other not? One prayed with his whole heart and was therefore answered; the other did not pray with his whole heart and was not answered. R. Eleazar, however, said: The one man was praying before his final sentence had been pronounced (in Heaven), the other after his final sentence had been pronounced. R. Isaac said: Supplication/crying out to God is good for a man whether before the final sentence had been pronounced or after.[32]

This honest exchange struggles to answer the $64,000 question of why some prayers get answered and others seem to have fallen on Deaf Divine Ears. Could it be the degree of sincerity? Or perhaps it is a matter of timing? Rabbi Isaac concludes the piece by pointing out that the subjective benefits of prayer are worthwhile, in any event; we humans need to give voice to our deepest sentiments, beliefs, needs, experiences.

In another Talmudic narrative, about Rabbi Hanina ben Dosa of the first century, the specific relationship of prayer to healing is touched upon:

Our Rabbis taught: Once the son of R. Gamliel fell ill. He (R. Gamliel) sent two scholars to R. Hanina ben Dosa to ask him to pray for him (for his son). When he (R. Hanina ben Dosa) saw them (the two scholars) he went to an upper chamber and prayed for him. When he came down he said to them (the two scholars): "Go, for the fever has left him." They (the two scholars) said to him (to R. Hanina ben Dosa): "Are you a prophet?" He said to them: "I am neither a prophet nor the son of a prophet, but I learned this from experience. *If my prayer is fluent in my mouth, I know that it is accepted; but if not, I know that it is rejected.*" They (the two scholars) sat down and made a note of the precise moment. When they came to R. Gamliel, he said to them: "By the Temple service! You have not been a moment too late or too soon, but so it happened: at that very moment the fever left him and he asked for water to drink."

On another occasion it happened that R. Hanina ben Dosa went to study Torah with R. Johanan ben Zakkai. The son of R. Johanan ben Zakkai fell ill. He (R. Johanan ben Zakkai) said to him: "Hanina my son, pray for him that he may live." He (R. Hanina) put his head between his knees and prayed for him, and he lived. Said R. Johanan ben Zakkai: "If ben Zakkai had stuck his head between his knees for the whole day, no notice would have been taken of him." Said his wife to him: "Is Hanina greater than you are!?" He replied to her: "No, but he is like a servant before the king, and I am like a nobleman before the king."[33]

The classic commentator Rashi explains that the servant is a *ben bayit*, a member of the household, who comes and goes without special permission, unlike the nobleman, who does not habitually come before him (and, indeed, much fanfare and fuss may accompany his visit). The implication seems to be that for the prayer to be efficacious, it needs to be a regular and fluent part of life.

"Theurgic" Prayer

In this connection, it is extremely important to note that Judaism discourages turning to prayer as one might to a vending machine:

Antignos of Socho received the tradition from Simon the Righteous, who used to say: Be not like the servants who serve the master on condition of receiving reward. Rather, be as servants who serve the master without the condition of receiving reward; and let the fear/awe of Heaven be upon you.[34]

Though one may certainly petition God in Judaism—throughout the day—and one is not forbidden to serve God with an expectation that one will be rewarded, the highest form of service is when one is inspired and motivated by love of God.[35]

Praying for "Healing into Death"

There are all kinds of dimensions to what we describe as "healing." A very potent story from the Talmud describes the often difficult, but necessary, transition from "Praying for Healing" to what might be called "Praying for Healing into Death." It describes the very challenging day on which Rabbi Judah the Prince, the second- /third-century redactor of the Mishnah (who was such a central leader that he is called simply "Rabbi") died:

On the day that Rabbi was dying, the Rabbis decreed a public fast and offered prayers for heavenly mercy. They, furthermore, announced that whoever said that Rabbi was dead would be stabbed with a sword. Rabbi's handmaid ascended the roof and prayed:

> "The immortals desire Rabbi to join them, and the mortals desire Rabbi to remain with them; may it be the will of God that the mortals may overpower the immortals."

When, however, she saw how often Rabbi resorted to the privy, painfully taking off his *tefillin* and putting them on again, she prayed:

> "May it be the will of the Almighty that the immortals may overpower the mortals."

As the Rabbis incessantly continued their prayers for heavenly mercy, she took up a jar and threw it down from the roof to the ground. For a moment they ceased praying, and the soul of Rabbi departed to its eternal rest.[36]

Like a hospice or palliative care team member, Rabbi's housekeeper is praiseworthy for her profound sensitivity to Rabbi's suffering and her ability to shift from the understandable desires of those who treasured him in this life, to his needs and the reality of his moving on. Prayer, when all is said and done, is not only about petition but about presence, mindfulness, gratitude, praise, and more—putting into words the numinous transitions of life.

"The Healing Package"

To adherents of some faiths, "faith" is deeply, almost exclusively associated with prayer, but Judaism has long maintained more of a "tripod" of foci, along the lines of this famous adage of Simon the Righteous (fourth century BCE): "The world stands on three things: On Torah, on Service of God (Prayer), and on Acts of Loving Kindness."[37]

From this one sentence, we can summarize what life requires, and certainly what a response to suffering demands: Torah, prayer, and deeds of lovingkindness.

Though Judaism did not, over the millennia, develop its own medical science, it did have a lot to say to those who seek to cure and to heal. Maimonides is certainly the "go-to guy" in this regard. Interestingly, when confronted with the theological question of how/why physicians are allowed to heal others when God has seen fit to inflict suffering on people, he did not turn to the biblical text that other authorities had utilized before.[38] Strikingly, Maimonides, instead, draws on this biblical commandment:

> If you see your fellow's ox or sheep gone astray, do not ignore it; you must take it back to your fellow. If your fellow does not live near you or you do not know who he is, you shall bring it home and it shall remain with you until your fellow claims it; then *you shall restore it to him* [Emphasis added]. You shall do the same with his ass; you shall do the same with his garment; and so too shall you do with anything that your fellow loses and you find: you may not hide yourself. . . .[39]

Maimonides uses this as the basis of a binding religious obligation to render medical care: "It is obligatory from the Torah for the physician to heal the sick and this is included in the explanation of the scriptural phrase *and you shall restore it to him*, meaning to heal his body."[40]

So, to Maimonides, the enterprise of healing can be derived from the biblical obligation of *hashavat aveidot*, "restoring something lost"—a provocative metaphor and compelling encapsulation of what it is to minister to those who suffer, whether medically, spiritually, psychologically, socially, etc. Maimonides, indeed, could be said to have maintained quite a holistic approach to the human being; as Joel Kraemer writes, "Maimonides made the interdependence of body and soul a primary rule of therapeutics."[41] Maimonides advises doctors accordingly: "In order to strengthen the vital powers, one should employ musical instruments and tell patients gay stories which will make his heart swell and narratives that will distract the mind and cause them and their friends to laugh."[42]

The physician should have both technical knowledge and skill as well as understand the patient's personality and lifestyle: Maimonides cited Galen as saying that in deciding on a treatment the physician needs to observe seven things: "... the nature of the sickness, the nature of the patient, his age, his habits, the nature of the town, the season of the year, and the constitution of the surrounding air."[43]

Summarizing: The Portals and Resources of Community and Tradition

In sum, Jewish approaches to those who suffer are based on Judaism's ancient holistic appreciation that human beings have many interacting dimensions—among them, the physiological, emotional, psychological, social, and spiritual. Health and healing depend on the interrelationship of Body, Mind, and Spirit—one might say, on reaching in, reaching out, and reaching up. The axes of community and tradition are essential components in life in general and in healing in particular.

SEVEN QUESTIONS FOR RESEARCH STUDY

Given all of the above, this writer is compelled to propose the following areas for inquiry and research. In doing so, I do not expect that all are easily designed studies, and some may turn out to be all but impossible to execute. But these seven questions remain of interest to this Jewish mind:

1. What is the relative healing potential and place of each member of the "Team": clergy, educators, musicians and artists, medical professionals, psychotherapists, *bikkur cholim* ("visiting the sick") volunteers, etc.? What can each contribute and how? How might they form the desired positively impactful team? Are certain medical issues/challenges (heart disease, Parkinson's, MS, etc.) better addressed by different parties in the team?
2. How *does* Torah heal? What sources and formats of Torah study might be said to contribute to healing? For example, what is the healing potential of Talmudic study as compared to Midrashic

exploration, or delving into the Five Books of Moses as compared to investigating Psalms? How does individual Torah study compare to having a regular study partner, or being a part of a committed study group, in healing impact?

3. Evaluate key psychospiritual challenges and resources and their impacts on health. Study these poles/themes: shame/image of God, hope/despair, guilt/responsibility, forgiveness/blame, chaos/meaningfulness, and perhaps one or two more.
4. How does the self-concept of the healer influence outcomes? For example, if s/he sees him/herself as restorer of something lost, or repairer of something broken, or warrior-chief, or choreographer/orchestra leader, or guide/leader—are there different health implications? How might/does this impact on the curative or healing journey?
5. Related to question 4, does/can the spiritual life of the healer contribute to physiological outcomes? For example, if the healer engages in prayer, with or without patients—or if s/he struggles with spiritual issues by engaging in studying layers of texts, perhaps with a partner, does it impact patients' well-being? What, how, and when?
6. "Mutual weeping" was touched on as a kind of "Jewish healing intervention," but this runs against the grain of much of contemporary health professional culture and training. If healers were not only allowed but encouraged to relate to patients on an emotional plane, and to express their emotional connections openly and deeply, what might be the health implications for those patients?
7. The Jewish year has a rhythm of markers—weekly Torah portions, new moons, holidays, fast days, etc. The Jewish calendar has a flow of themes and foci (for example, from slavery to freedom; change and repentance; coping with vulnerability; etc.), and a range of rituals and practices (constructing/

inhabiting a hut for a week, dramatically altering diet for a week, raucous celebrations, etc.). What health/healing resources can be described, evaluated, and projected from this repertoire?

IF YOU THINK IT WAS HARD TO BEGIN ...

Our subject is vast, and our journey on these pages has not exhausted the subject. It seems that concluding is nearly as challenging as beginning! But the following Hasidic teaching on the words of Abraham in Genesis 18:27—"I am but dust and ashes"—will help us bring this to a close; note how it utilizes the end of the text with which we began, concerning the Divine Image:

Everyone must have two pockets, so that s/he can reach into the one or the other, according to his/her needs: In the right pocket are to be the words: "For my sake was the world created" [M. *Sanhedrin* 4:5] and in the left: "I am dust and ashes [Genesis 18:27]."[44]

In the end, when all is said and done, how we relate to illness and suffering, or health and well-being, is about how we navigate mortality and life itself. We are, indeed, but dust and ashes, but we are, at the very same time, each of us, an entire Universe.

NOTES

1. Paraphrased from Zohar *Devarim* 299b.
2. Tosafot *Ta'anit* 10b.
3. Genesis 1:27.
4. M. *Sanhedrin* 4:5.
5. Paraphrased from Sa'adia Gaon's philosophic classic, *Emunot v'Deot* [Egypt, 933], 4:1–2.
6. Judah Loew, *Sefer Derech HaHayim* [1589] (Tel Aviv, Israel: Sinai Pub., 1954), cited in Joseph L. Baron, ed., *A Treasury of Jewish Quotations* [1956] (New York: Jason Aronson, 1985), 196.
7. Abraham Joshua Heschel, "Symbolism and Jewish Faith" [1954], in *Moral Grandeur and Spiritual Audacity*, ed. Susannah Heschel (New York: Farrar, Straus, and Giroux, 1996), 80–99, quotation on 84.

8. Attributed to Menachem Mendel Schneerson, seventh leader of the Chabad-Lubavitch dynasty, accessed at http://www.chabad.org/therebbe/article_cdo/aid/60872/jewish/Power-of-the-Individual.htm.

9. R. Pinhas of Koretz, *Nofet Tzufim* (Warsaw, 1929), 59.

10. *Berakhot* 10a.

11. Paraphrased from *Sifre* Deuteronomy 306.

12. *Sanhedrin* 91a–b.

13. Translation is my own; the *Mi Sheberakh* can be found in most Jewish prayer books.

14. Leviticus *Rabbah, Parashat Behar* 34:3.

15. Quoted from Philo Judaeus, "The Worse Attacks the Better" section 10, cited in Michael Strassfield, *A Book of Life: Embracing Judaism as a Spiritual Practice* [2002] (Woodstock, VT: Jewish Lights, 2006), 7.

16. Samson Raphael Hirsch, "Eleventh Letter," in *The Nineteen Letters of Ben Uziel: Being a Spiritual Presentation of the Principles of Judaism* [1836], trans. Bernard Drachman (New York: Funk & Wagnalls, 1899), 107–12, quotation on 112.

17. Deuteronomy 5:2ff.

18. From Midrash *Tanhuma* (Buber recension) [1885], *Parashat Nitzavim* 8, 25b, cited in Baron, *A Treasury of Jewish Quotations*, 70.

19. *Sotah* 14a.

20. From Maimonides, *Mishneh Torah: Laws Concerning Moral Dispositions and Ethical Conduct* [c. 1170–80], cited in Jessica Gribetz, *Wise Words: Jewish Thoughts and Stories Through the Ages* (New York: HarperCollins, 1997), 135.

21. From Isaac Arama, *Akedat Yitzhak* [1522], *Sha'ar* xxvi, cited in Simkha Y. Weintraub, "Some Jewish Quotes From Over the Centuries Related to Bodily Health," Jewish Board of Family and Children's Services, 2009, accessed at http://www.jcprograms.org/documents/BodilyHealthQuotes.pdf.

22. Paraphrased from "The First Gate: The Gate of Pride," in *Orchot Tzaddikim* [1581]; for a recent English translation of the entire volume, see *Orchot Tzaddikim,* ed. Gavriel Zaloshinsky, trans. Shraga Silverstein (Jerusalem: Feldheim Publishers, 1995), 35–37.

23. From Ba'al Shem Tov, as brought forth in *Keter Shem Tov: Anthology of Teachings of R. Israel Baal Shem Tov*, ed. Aaron of Apt (Brooklyn: Kehot, 1987), 4a, cited in Gribetz, *Wise Words*, 135.

24. *Berakhot* 5b.

25. Many have noted that the metaphor of prison seems unfair and unhelpful regarding illness—in that we do not want to suggest that suffering is a punishment for misdeeds. This would need a broader discussion, but for now, suffice it to say, as many individuals who are suffering have, that "it sure feels like a punishment."

26. Tsvi Blanchard, "To Join Heaven and Earth: Maimonides and the Laws of Bikkur Cholim," *The Outstretched Arm* 4, no. 1 (Fall 1994), accessed at http://www.ncjh.org/downloads/BikurJoinHeavenEarth.doc.

27. *Ketubot* 77b; note that this section of Proverbs was understood to be talking about the Torah.

28. M. *Avot* 2:7.

29. *Eruvin* 54a.

30. *Song of Songs Rabbah* 2:46.

31. Which brings to mind recent studies that show that placebos seem to be most effective when there is a trusting relationship between patient and doctor.

32. *Rosh HaShannah* 18a.

33. *Berakhot* 34b.

34. M. *Avot* 1:3.

35. Rabbi Dr. Joseph Soloveitchik, arguably the greatest mind of twentieth-century Orthodoxy, taught, in effect, that "it is the duty of the Jew to cry out to God in times of trouble." See Joseph B. Soloveitchik, *Shiurim le-Zecher Avi Mori* (Jerusalem: Akiva Yosef, 1983).

36. *Ketubot* 104a.

37. M. *Avot* 1:2.

38. Exodus 21:19.

39. Deuteronomy 22:1–3.

40. From Moses Maimonides, *Commentary on the Mishnah, Nedarim* 4:4, as cited in Fred Rosner, *Contemporary Biomedical Ethical Issues and Jewish Law* (Jersey City, NJ: Ktav, 2007), 165. See also *Shulchan Arukh, Yoreh De'ah* 336.

41. Joel L. Kraemer, *Maimonides: The Life and World of One of Civilization's Greatest Minds* (New York: Doubleday, 2008), 462.

42. From Moses Maimonides, *The Preservation of Youth: Essays on Health*, trans. Hirsch L. Gordon (New York: Philosophical Library, 1958), cited in Union for Reform Judaism, "Jewish Texts," *Health Care for All*, accessed at http://urj.org//socialaction/issues/healthcare//?syspage=article&item_id=1836.

43. Moses Maimonides, *The Art of Cure (Extracts from Galen)*, ed. and trans. Uriel S. Barzel (Haifa, Israel: Maimonides Research Institute, 1992), 108, cited in Moses Maimonides, *On Asthma*, ed. and trans. Gerrit Bos (Chicago: University of Chicago Press, 2001), 123.

44. Martin Buber, *Ten Rungs: Collected Hasidic Sayings* [1947] (New York: Citadel Press, 1995), 106.

PART 2

CHRISTIAN PERSPECTIVES

THE CHAPTERS in this second section of *Healing to All Their Flesh* concern themselves with the broad interface of the Christian religion with the kinds of concepts and issues that animate biomedical and health-focused research—an enterprise that essentially defines the contemporary religion and health field. The authors, all theological scholars, approach this topic from different angles, yet share a common tack: each provides a passionate and uncompromising critique of existing streams of research and writing in this field and each, in turn, offers creatively idealized alternatives to which researchers in this field would be wise to pay heed. As with the rabbinic authors in Part 1, these contributors represent a diversity of denominational streams, as well as intellectual traditions.

Warren Kinghorn provides a masterful analysis of the inherent limitations of empirical research, the study of health, and the concept of religion and details the promise of a science of human flourishing, all from a perspective richly informed by Aquinas' *Summa theologiae*. Therese Lysaught expertly dissects the study of spirituality within medicine, identifying it as a biopolitically constructed discourse that reinforces a particularly dualistic worldview about the human body and about health. Stephen Post introduces the concept of the Ontological Generality as a theological framework to interpret the relation between religion and health, drawing on the example of Alcoholics Anonymous and discussing existing research in the context of divine love. John Swinton's chapter is the most constructively conceptual in this book: he asks us to reconsider what we mean by religion (and wonders why Jesus never seems to be part of this discussion) and how we define and study health (which suffers from an implicit positivism and which would benefit by replacement with *shalom*). Stanley Hauerwas takes a look back at his celebrated *Suffering Presence*, a quarter century after its publication, revisiting themes related to the body, the patient role, and the conflicting medical and Christian perspectives on both.

In reading these chapters, one is struck by how they distinctively contrast, on the whole, with the Jewish contributions in Part 1. For the rabbinic authors, the idea of an interconnection or relation among spirituality, theology, and health is tacit. The great rabbinic sages wrote extensively on such issues, and there is enough material on this theme in the Jewish canon to fill many volumes. Our five rabbis, accordingly, focus their efforts on more practical exercises in translating rabbinic perspectives into guidance for real-world concerns: e.g., patienthood, aging, bioethics, healing, and so on. The relation itself is not intrinsically problematic for them, but how to make sense of it, how to apply it to one's life, what to do with this observation is a vital, pressing, and significant issue.

For the Christian theologians in Part 2, this relation is indeed quite problematic, and so we are treated to a set of incisive dissertations pointing out conceptual and theoretical concerns with the field and providing guidance on how to work through or around them. The idea of a field of empirical research on this subject—as well as the current state of said field—is concerning specifically because of its ongoing failure to engage profound definitional issues. For the rabbinic contributors, the idea of such a field is not problematic on these grounds, in and of itself, and, indeed, little is stated directly about said "field." The main issue is that scholars have not been asking the right questions, nor are the right applications being made (i.e., to the doctor-patient relationship, to senescence, to spiritual development, to medical ethics decision making, to God-centered healing, etc.). Accordingly, they offer a brand-new roadmap, reflecting the historic rabbinic emphasis on praxis over theory. The Christian authors, by contrast, in the chapters that follow, offer a deeply theologically moored critique of the very underpinnings of the religion and health field, reflecting distinct intellectual traditions and, like a laser, focusing in on conceptual and theoretical deficiencies that require addressing in order for the field to right itself and flourish.

WARREN KINGHORN

6. ST. THOMAS AQUINAS AND THE END(S) OF RELIGION, SPIRITUALITY, AND HEALTH

Et precor te, ut ad illud ineffabile convivium
me peccatorem perducere digneris,
ubi tu cum Filio tuo
et Spiritu Sancto.
Sanctis tuis es
lux vera
satietas plena,
gaudium sempiternum,
jucunditas consummata,
et felicitas perfecta.
Per eundem Christum Dominum nostrum.
Amen.

I also pray that You bring me, a sinner
to that ineffable banquet where You dwell
with your Son
and Holy Spirit.
You Who are for Your saints
true light,
complete fulfillment,
eternal joy,
consummate delight,
and perfect happiness.
Through the same Christ our Lord,
Amen.[1]

The principal problems with the field of "religion, spirituality, and health," from a Christian theological perspective, are, respectively, "religion," "spirituality," and "health." Each of these concepts, that is to say, resists the kind of stipulative definition that is critical for the design and conduct of an empirical research program; when modern-day empirical researchers propose such definitions, they rarely acknowledge the complex history of these terms within the history of Christian thought and practice. It is common, for example, for interpreters and authors within the "religion and health" literature to offer definitions for "religion" and "spirituality" that distinguish these from each other: "religion" is generally associated with institutions ("organized religion") and public and/or ritual practices, whereas "spirituality" is frequently taken to denote some form of private experience or contact with the divine that is not essentially related to religious institutions or public observances.[2] This distinction clearly names the way that many people (particularly, though not exclusively, affluent, nonminority, North Atlantic people) think and speak about these terms, but as a general account of the use of these terms, either historically or in the present, it fails. As Wuthnow,[3] Carrette and King,[4] and others have demonstrated, the divorce of "spirituality" from "religion" is a late twentieth-century American and European development, reflective of a culture of increasing individualism and resistance to religious or political authority. The individualistic concept of spirituality may apply imperfectly, for example, to the experience of many African-Americans,[5] and as a Euro-Christian construct, "spirituality" may paradoxically exclude and marginalize racial and ethnic minorities.[6] Certainly, Christians of earlier centuries would generally not have thought it possible to be "spiritual but not religious." But "religion" too, as it is used in the "religion and health" scholarship, turns out to be historically and culturally constructed.

Nicholas Lash, for instance, persuasively argues that "religion," as a description of a component of human life and culture comprising specific traditions such as Judaism, Christianity, and Islam, was a European invention for a colonializing culture that needed "new instruments for [the] conceptual mapping and control" of the rapidly expanding known world; "religion" became, in this context, "a science that has an unequivocal language with which it speaks and uniform objects of which it speaks" to describe a world "made of one kind of stuff and driven by one set of forces."[7] Joel Shuman and Keith Meador, in what is still the most sustained and careful theological critique of the "'contemporary rapprochement' between medicine and religion,"[8] argue that "religion" has been both subsumed into and produced by a capitalist logic of exchange, such that both "spirituality" and "religion" are "transformed by the market into means, among others, of achieving a better life now."[9] One aspect of this "better life now" is certainly "health," which Shuman and Meador argue has been sundered from its properly communal and participatory context and has become "fetishized," pursued and exchanged "without reference to the persons or communities who produce it or to its proper place in a hierarchy of the goods of a society committed to pursuing a substantive account of human flourishing."[10] They might have noted that "health" as a concept is a perfect candidate for this sort of commodification, since it is a concept of immense social power (the ostensible goal of the "health care disciplines") that hardly anyone, including medical practitioners, ever bothers to define. When careful attention is given to proposed definitions of "health," the concept turns out to be slippery and controversial,[11] with the ironic result that clinicians and patients who promote and seek "health" can only rarely articulate what, exactly, they are promoting and seeking. "Health" provides the perfect modern teleology, capable of serving as a potent (if elusive) final end in a culture that thinks that it has long moved past the need for final ends.

If in fact it is true that "religion," "spirituality," and "health" are all contested and socially constructed concepts that elude the working definitions assigned to them by "religion and health" researchers, this presents a significant and structural problem for the field, both in the way that research questions are framed and asked and in the interpretation of research results. Many important and interesting research findings of the past three decades—the finding that religious service attendance correlates with lower use of hospital services, for example,[12] or that measurable patterns of positive or negative religious coping are associated with response to trauma and serious illness[13]—are still valid and useful, but it is nonetheless the case that many contemporary research instruments and designs bear the marks of contested and culturally relative assumptions that then produce research results and interpretations that reinforce (without testing or contesting) these problematic, culturally relative assumptions.

For example, the Functional Assessment of Chronic Illness Therapy-Spiritual Well-Being scale (FACIT-Sp) is a well-designed psychometric instrument specifically designed to measure "spirituality" rather than "religion" in persons with chronic illness. Items (rated on a five-point continuum) include, "I feel a sense of purpose in my life" and "I know that whatever happens with my illness, things will be okay."[14] In the decade since its introduction, the FACIT-Sp has been used in a number of clinical trials, giving rise to claims that various interventions "improve the spiritual well-being" of certain patient populations.[15] Ando, Morita, Akechi, and Okamoto,[16] for example, administered a brief intervention titled the Short-Term Life Review to a randomized subsample of sixty-eight terminally ill Japanese cancer patients; in this two-session intervention, patients were asked to reflect on questions such as, "What is the most important thing in your life and why?" and were then presented with an album, compiled by the therapist, in which responses were decorated with drawings and photographs. Compared to control subjects who received an equivalent amount of supportive care, patients randomized to the Short-Term Life Review reported significantly higher (i.e., better) scores on the FACIT-Sp, lower levels of self-reported anxiety and depression, and a significantly lower endorsement of the statement, "I am distressed that I am being a burden to family members," among other items.

The results of this well-executed study—and many others like it—are a contribution to the clinical literature on care at the end of life; in the context of modern biomedicine, it is a welcome and good reminder that time and space for simple, human questions such as these can perhaps do more to reduce existential suffering than many other high-tech, expensive interventions. But it remains the fact, from a Christian theological perspective, that there is no clear reason, beyond an arbitrary convention of naming, why such improvement should be labeled "spiritual," as opposed, for example, to "holistic," "narrative," or "existential." At the very least, insofar as the well-being promoted in this study is referred to as "spiritual well-being," it reinforces the common (and contested) presumptions that "spirituality" is not essentially connected to any religious tradition or to any particular understanding of God; that it inheres in individuals, not communities or cultures;

that it can be the subject of technical modification and can, therefore, be enhanced by some form of commercially available instrument; and that spiritual well-being can be effected individually or dyadically, rather than communally. For researchers working within the structural and liberal constraints of modern biomedical institutions, such presumptions might be unavoidable; but as Shuman and Meador argue persuasively, for Christians and Christian communities to internalize them would be poisonous. It would be a great shame, for example, if deference to the biomedical model led Christian communities to cede "spiritual care" in end-of-life situations to professional chaplains and mental health clinicians, thereby reneging on their own communal obligations to dying persons and, even more, to attention to the social and structural sins that precipitate the loneliness and isolation that interventions like the Short-Term Life Review are designed to treat.

From the perspective of Christian theology, what is needed within the "religion, spirituality, and health" movement is not more or better empirical research, nor the abolition of such research, but rather the ongoing development of theologically informed *theoretical* models that avoid the conceptual shortcomings of "religion," "spirituality," and "health." Such models, if successful, would *enhance* and *improve* empirical investigation into the relationship between faithfulness and human flourishing by providing fruitful imaginative resources for the design of research questions and for the interpretation of the results of new and existing research. Any successful model would, on a formal level, display certain attributes. First, it would provide a way to narrate the relationship of "health" (including health of the body and "mental health") to Christian theological conceptions of human flourishing such as salvation and sanctification. Second, and related to this, it would provide a way to narrate the relationship between the body and the "soul" or "spirit" and, correlatively, the relationship between the "physical" and the "spiritual." Third, it would set boundaries for the concepts of "religion" and "spirituality" and would narrate how each of these relate to each other, to the moral life, to the life of the body, and to the pursuit of the good life. Fourth (and finally), it would illumine ways in which the empirical methods of the biological and social sciences might bear fruitful and faithful results, and also the limits of this mode of investigation.

There are likely many instances, in the long history of Christian tradition, which would satisfy these criteria; Shuman and Meador,[17] for example, fruitfully explore the contemporary work of Karl Barth and Wendell Berry. In this essay, however, I turn to the anthropology and moral psychology of St. Thomas Aquinas (1225–1274). Aquinas might seem anachronistic to some because he lived and wrote prior to the advent of modern empirical science or modern political liberalism; but precisely *because* of this, his system of thought can be helpful in liberating researchers and clinicians from the problematic assumptions that both empirical science and political liberalism entail. In what follows, I do not intend to trace in detail the complex and sometimes difficult contours of Aquinas' psychology. Rather, I will briefly and sometimes schematically draw on Aquinas' work, particularly as expressed in its most mature form in the *Summa theologiae*, to imagine a new paradigm within which empirical work on "religion, spirituality, and health" might be conceived. Such an account will not answer all questions but will, I hope, create a fruitful space within which further questions can be raised.[18]

AQUINAS ON EMPIRICAL SCIENCE (AND ITS LIMITS)

Aquinas' work can be conceptually fruitful for the modern "religion, spirituality, and health" movement in large part because of its congeniality to it. In our own time, if he is considered at all, Aquinas is often dismissed as a "scholastic," preoccupied with the provability of God's existence or with abstract metaphysical questions. But in the philosophical and theological culture of the thirteenth century, Aquinas stood out for his emphasis on the utility of empirical investigation into the material world (including the material of the human person) and for his insistence on the importance of the senses for human knowledge, including intellectual knowledge.[19] Whereas major Christian theologians in the centuries prior to Aquinas such as Anselm of

Canterbury and Hugh of St. Victor were careful not to disparage the goodness of the material world, they inherited from Plato, via Augustine of Hippo, a focus on introspection and rational investigation as a mode for the discovery of truth. This introspective mode did not preclude or censor empirical observation of the natural world, but neither did it do much to encourage it.

In the Western Europe of the twelfth and thirteenth centuries, however, much was changing. Increased trade and contact with non-Western cultures had allowed multiple texts of Aristotle, lost for centuries to the Latin West but preserved in the Muslim cultures of the Middle East and Spain, to be reintroduced to Western philosophical thought and to be translated into Latin, along with the Aristotelian commentaries of the Islamic scholars Ibn Sina (Avicenna) and Ibn Roschd (Averroes) as well as the work of the Jewish rabbi/physician/philosopher Moses Maimonides. With Aristotle and his commentators came increased attention to the close empirical observation of the world that Aristotle had championed in his own time (i.e., *De Partibus Animalium*), such that the Western intellectual polymath Albert the Great (ca. 1193–1280) distinguished himself not only in his theological work but also in his works of botany and zoology.[20] Albert became Thomas Aquinas' teacher, and although Aquinas never himself wrote works of empirical science or natural philosophy, his work displays a deep respect for the goodness and integrity of the natural world and for the importance of sensory observation. The intellectual faculty of the soul and its knowledge, Aquinas held, are immaterial,[21] but the data for this knowledge is *acquired* not immaterially but by way of the senses, as the senses receive into themselves the forms of objects of sensation and as embodied perceptual mechanisms represent the sensed object as an internal image, or phantasm, from which the intellect can then abstract the immaterial form of the thing.[22] This perceptual theory of Aquinas is remarkable both for its content and for its form. In its content, it displays Aquinas' conviction that disciplined observation and reflection on material reality (i.e., empirical methodology) is important for proper knowledge of the world. In its form, it shows how Aquinas, in his theological anthropology, incorporated what was at that time the cutting-edge scientific psychology of his time (that of Aristotle and his commentators) into the core of his theory. Aquinas' respect for empiricism also displays itself in his consistent and generally uncritical use of the generally accepted pathophysiological theory of his time, the four-humor theory, in his theory of the emotions and in his moral psychology.[23] Had the (somewhat dubious) term existed in his own day, Aquinas would surely be credited with doing "neurotheology."

All of this is not to say, however, that Aquinas placed absolute trust either in sense-knowledge or in natural human reason. He was too aware of the fallibility of human sensation and human reason, and—significantly—of his intellectual and spiritual debt to the received Christian tradition that he took such great care to transmit fairly and faithfully. In the very first question of the *Summa theologiae* he considers, in characteristic *disputatio* format, whether any further doctrine is required besides philosophy (which, at that time, would have included all of the "sciences"). His answer is an unequivocal "yes," for two reasons. First, he argues, the end to which humans are ultimately directed—God—cannot be known by human reason (or observation) alone, and because human salvation depends on recognition of this end, "it was necessary for [human] salvation that certain truths which exceed human reason should be made known . . . by divine revelation."[24] But he follows this by arguing that divine revelation is necessary even for truths about God that *could* be known by human reason, "because the truth about God such as reason could discover, would only be known by a few, and that after a long time, and with the admixture of many errors."[25]

Aquinas' treatment of the limited goodness of the empirical sciences bears several lessons for the contemporary "religion, spirituality, and health" movement. First, in his example, Aquinas demonstrates that investigation of the material and psychological aspects of religious belief and practice, together with investigation of the material and psychological sequelae of such belief and practice, can find an honorable place in the work of Christian scholarship. Aquinas' moral psychology, particularly his detailed treatments of human action,[26] of the emotions/"passions,"[27] and of habit,[28] are so contextually integrated into his moral theology that any distinction between the two is problematically arbitrary. But Aquinas would want to be very careful about the extent to which the results of empirical investigation are used to make categorical or essential claims about their subject matter. The fact that one has analyzed religious belief and practice as material and psychological phenomena does not mean that one has thereby discovered anything essential about "religion," "spirituality," or "health" (including that they exist); it means only that one has analyzed religious belief and practice as material and psychological phenomena. For Aquinas, such observations can be correctly named and interpreted only when they are placed into the larger teleological and conceptual context of the revealed Christian story, which cannot itself be reduced to the psychological or accounted for through empirical methods alone.

AQUINAS ON HEALTH (AND ITS LIMITS)

"Health" plays a powerful and odd role in the logic and practice of modern biomedicine. Along with its cognate "healthy," it dominates medical language ("health care," "health professionals," etc.) and serves as the presumptive end toward which all medical practice strives—but it is a remarkably *unarticulated* end. Most people agree that health is somehow the absence of or relative freedom from "disease" or "illness," such that to be "healed" from disease is, somehow, to embody better health; but relatively few contemporary clinicians and researchers ever bother to articulate what "health" positively entails, apart from the absence of disease. The well-known World Health Organization definition, which states that health "is a state of complete physical, mental, and social well-being and not merely the absence of disease or infirmity,"[29] seems too broad in that any lack of well-being is therefore understood as "unhealthy," and there is no specification of *who decides* what constitutes "well-being." Such a definition begs the question, without resolution, about what relationship medicine should have with the pursuit of "health."[30] But despite much debate, no alternative positive account of "health" has ever gained wide acceptance within biomedicine. Instead, "health" is often invoked but rarely defended, and the biomedical culture, by colluding in this, enables "health" to function as a kind of shadow teleology, enabling modern researchers and clinicians (and patients) to *act* for an end without the troublesome burden of *justifying* or *defending* that end. Such a collusion is convenient for the biomedical culture but is dangerous for everyone else, in that "health" can borrow the cultural and scientific prestige of modern medicine to set ends that would, under any other name, be more contested.[31]

Aquinas would have wanted nothing to do with any of this. Rooted as he was in a medieval philosophical culture inherited from Plato, Aristotle, and Augustine (and many like-minded others), Aquinas understood that the first task of any practical activity is to identify its end, such that "final cause" plays at least as important a role in his thought as "material cause" or "efficient cause." And the end of human life, for Aquinas, was not bodily health (*sanitas*) but beatitude (*beatitudo*), the doxological union of the human with the One who is the end of all human striving. *Beatitudo* is often rendered as "happiness" in English translations of Aquinas, and might also be fruitfully rendered "human flourishing," as it is closely related to Aristotle's *eudaimonia*. Indeed, *beatitudo* does entail, for Aquinas, nearly everything that Aristotle intended by the Greek term *eudaimonia*: an integrated human life in which the enlivened body, habituated through teaching and practice to desire what is life-giving and to shun what is harmful, displays through wise embodied practice a life that is mature and harmoniously satisfying and that contributes to the flourishing of the community of which it is a part. Embodied actualized dispositions, or habits, which when displayed contribute to the flourishing of the individual and of the community are known as virtues; embodied actualized dispositions which, when displayed, harm the individual or community, are known as vices. But unlike Aristotle, for whom the norm of virtue was the flourishing of the Greek *polis* (i.e., the Athenian city-state), for Aquinas the norm of virtue was the *ratio*, or reason, of the triune God; as for Augustine, the most important *polis* for Aquinas was not Athens, or Rome or Paris, nor even the church of his day, but rather the *civitas Dei*, bound not by common temporal or even ecclesiastical rulers but by a common love for God and the things of God.[32]

Though Aquinas was a political realist and had much to say about the way that the political and ecclesiastical rulers of his day should conduct themselves, he makes clear that human happiness (*beatitudo*) consists ultimately not in wealth, not in honors, not in fame or glory, not in power, not in any bodily good, not in pleasure, not even in the work of philosophy, but only in the vision of God, in which all human desires come to an active and lively rest in the One who is alone able to fulfill them.[33] Such vision is not a simple matter; it requires that one not be so preoccupied by the pursuit of limited pleasures in mutable things that one misses the less titillating, but infinitely more satisfying, things of God; it requires a will shaped to love things that are truly lovely and beautiful, instead of those things that only appear so.[34] In the conditions of embodied life, it requires also a body formed and habituated in the right patterns of desire, since (as above) the body is integral to the function of the embodied soul.[35] Such a well-formed life might seem elusive and unattainable, and indeed, for Aquinas, it is: like Augustine and unlike Aristotle, the Christian Aquinas believed that humans, stained by sin, could never attain genuine happiness on their own, even in the best of circumstances. A prior action of God is required, a divine love that comes graciously to humans and that, through participation, enables the return of that love and the right ordering of desire. Such love, made possible through the work of Christ, Aquinas labeled *caritas*, charity; and insofar as *caritas* clearly names God as the ultimate end of human flourishing, toward which all of the other virtues (such as courage, temperance, and justice) are directed, *caritas* is for Aquinas the "form" of all of the other virtues.[36]

Aquinas' persistent insistence that happiness is to be found ultimately not in temporal or mutable goods but only in God means that all of his detailed moral psychology must be considered in theocentric perspective. This is not to say that he talks about God all the time in his work, even in the *Summa theologiae*; indeed, he clearly does not. Read in abstraction from the overall structure of the *Summa*, his account of the human person and the relation of body to soul[37] and his accounts of the passions,[38] habits,[39] and virtues[40] show the marks of a ground-up Aristotelian method in which the body and the psychological functioning of the person each have a "natural" integrity, including the capacity to acquire and display certain virtues, which does not depend on any conscious orientation to God or on any divinely "infused" virtue.[41] (One wonders whether Aquinas' relatively generous account of the human capacity for virtue apart from the confession of Christian faith was due to his own recognition of his debt to the Jewish and Islamic scholars through whom, in part, he had learned Aristotle.) This close-to-the-ground method, as stated above, rendered Aquinas very attentive and sympathetic to the medical and psychological sciences of his day, in ways that make him attractive to many modern-day theologians who are similarly attentive and sympathetic. But none of this changes the fundamental fact that for Aquinas no happiness is complete or fulfilled, short of God; no disposition of the body is ultimately life-giving if it does not aid the journey to God; no virtue is complete in itself, if it is not directed by divinely infused charity to supernatural ends.[42] For all of its immense Aristotelian complexity, then, the moral psychology of Aquinas merges seamlessly into his moral theology and demands a thoroughly teleological account of what it means to be human. The human is a *viator*, a wayfarer, journeying (back) to God, in whom alone the human can rest. Anything which aids or succors the *viator* on that journey is to be encouraged and promoted; anything which distracts or hinders the *viator* is to be shunned.

What is the role of bodily health (*sanitas*) in Aquinas' account of beatitude? Certainly, for Aquinas, bodily health is a blessing and a good to be pursued: Aquinas frequently commends attentive and responsible care of the body[43] and speaks favorably of the healing function of the medical arts of his day. The good of health, he writes, consists in a "certain commensuration of the humors in keeping with an animal's nature" and sickness (*aegritudo*) follows from disorder of the humors.[44] Medicine can be said to be the cause of health, and even to be "healthy" (*sanum*), because it restores this humoral balance.[45] Bodily health, then, is a good, a habit that disposes a body to be a functioning and *living* body, to do what bodies are supposed to do.[46] But it is remarkable, particularly in contrast to the conceptual dominance of "health" in our own day, how little attention Aquinas gives to *sanitas* in the *Summa theologiae*. He mentions it only a handful of times, often by way of example, and never devotes sustained argument to its nature or attainment. Furthermore, it is not at all clear in the *Summa theologiae* how one recognizes *sanitas* when it exists, except by recourse to broader criteria of judgment.

To judge a body "healthy," he argues, one needs to know its nature; but a body's "nature" is known only in its *act*, in what it does and how it functions. A body that functions well—as bodies ought to function—can, in that light, be called "healthy": quoting Aristotle, Aquinas writes that "man, or one of his members, is called healthy, when he can perform the operation of a healthy man."[47] The problem with this is that when one begins to speak of "the operation of a healthy man" as the comparative reference for "health," one begs the question as to what exactly that operation looks like; and the logic of Aquinas' system is that such "healthy" operation would be the life of virtue. It turns out, then, that Aquinas' *sanitas* is probably no more successful than modern concepts of "health" at defining the nature and meaning of bodily health without recourse to larger teleological considerations. Aquinas' distinct advantage, though, is that he does not need it to do so: because he has gone to such great lengths to establish what the final end of human life is (*beatitudo*), he is able to allow bodily health (*sanitas*) to remain an important but limited good that is known only in light of larger considerations and that comfortably and humbly occupies its subservient place in the ordering of proper human goods. He did not need (as we do) for "health" to fill a gaping teleological vacuum, because for him no such vacuum existed.

What lessons might Aquinas' treatment of *beatitudo* and *sanitas* have for the modern "religion, spirituality, and health" movement?

I suspect that were Aquinas listening to modern-day conversations about "health," he would want those who use the term to clarify whether by "health" they mean bodily health *(sanitas)* or whether they mean something closer to *eudaimonia* or even *beatitudo*. In some cases (e.g., public health campaigns to prevent malaria or HIV infection), he would clearly recognize his own concept of *sanitas*; in others (e.g., discussions about certain forms of "mental health," or "healthy lifestyles," or "spiritual fitness"), he would recognize a grasping approximation of *beatitudo*. In cases where *sanitas* is intended, Aquinas would likely applaud efforts to promote and foster this sort of "health" but would want to remind everyone that *sanitas* is a limited, proximate end in the larger context of human life; he would also probably find it interesting and a bit counterintuitive that anyone would want to think of religious devotional practices as a way to obtain *sanitas*, since such practices are properly instrumental not to *sanitas* but to the higher, more important end of *beatitudo*. He might even wonder aloud whether *sanitas* might be taking on too much teleological weight. On the other hand, in cases where "health" is used to refer to something like *beatitudo*, Aquinas would encourage those who use the term in this way to fully own the teleological import of this use, and would likely shake his head mournfully upon learning that many modern humans consider the wisest guides for the attainment of *beatitudo* to be not priests or theologians, nor even philosophers, but rather the practitioners of the medical and healing arts. But he would think it perfectly appropriate to consider religious devotional practices as instrumental for this form of "health"; as we will examine in the next section, that is precisely what these practices are for.

A final point about Aquinas' treatment of "health" before moving on to the contested terrain of "religion" and "spirituality": it is tempting to think of Aquinas' concept of bodily health (*sanitas*) as "physical" and his account of happiness (*beatitudo*) as "spiritual," given the theological and theocentric frame in which the latter takes its form. There is indeed some logic for this argument within Aquinas' system: *sanitas*, the proper disposition of the human body to its form, can be considered without specific reference to the truths of faith, to God, or to the infused virtues (even if, as above, it beckons toward them); whereas *beatitudo* terminates in the vision of God and cannot be considered apart from the God who makes it possible. Insofar, then, as *sanitas* is oriented to the proximate end of good bodily function and *beatitudo* is oriented toward supernatural ends (and dependent on the Spirit which, in Christian trinitarian doctrine, is the only proper referent of the "spiritual"), such a distinction is indeed plausible. But the fact that Aquinas distinguishes the "spiritual" from the "physical" does not mean that "spiritual" acts are wholly disembodied. The spiritual life of living humans, for Aquinas, is not some separate practical realm from the physical; it is simply the orientation of the living body (that is, the form-matter union of soul and body) to the things of the Spirit. Under the conditions of bodily life, the human journey to God is an embodied journey; it is precisely because the body is so essential to this journey that Aquinas gives such careful and detailed consideration to physiology and psychology. Despite his insistence on the immateriality of the intellectual faculty of the soul, Aquinas is not a proto-Cartesian substance dualist. Soul and body, for Aquinas, are united as form and matter, configuration to configured.[48] Human action, including "religious" action, is embodied action; human cognition, including cognition about "spiritual" things, is embodied cognition insofar as the intellect depends for its operation on the ongoing right-working of the embodied mechanisms of sensation and perception.[49] It would therefore come as no surprise to Aquinas, then, that "spiritual" practices have neurophysiological correlates,[50] or that religious devotional practices can change certain physiological parameters: to him, these findings, so striking in our day, would have only confirmed his Aristotelian (and non-Cartesian) anthropological assumptions.

AQUINAS ON RELIGION (AND ITS LIMITS), AND WHY SPIRITUALITY SHOULD BE ABOLISHED

So far we have considered ways that Aquinas' treatment of the empirical sciences and of "health" might bear fruit for theological analysis of the modern "religion, spirituality, and health" movement—but what, we might ask, of "religion" and "spirituality" themselves?

As with "health," any consideration of what Aquinas has to say about religion forces clarification about what one means by "religion." In the *Summa theologiae, religio* (religion) plays a limited but important role in Aquinas' theory of the virtues. He treats it as a virtue annexed to the cardinal moral virtue of justice; as justice is the rendering to another what he or she is due, so also religion is the rendering to God what God is due, though Aquinas is clear that this can never equal what is owed.[51] He approvingly quotes the pagan Cicero that "religion consists in offering service and ceremonial rites to a superior nature that men call divine," and he playfully considers whether the Latin word *religio* derives from *relego* ("to read again," as in "a religious man reads again those things which pertain to the worship of God"), *reeligo* ("to choose over again," as in "we ought to seek God again"), or *religo* ("to bind together," since religion binds individuals together in common worship). Whatever its proper etymology, Aquinas writes, God is the proper end of *religio,* since "it is He to Whom we ought to be bound as to our unfailing principle; to Whom also our choice should be resolutely directed as to our last end; and Whom we lose when we neglect Him by sin, and should recover by believing in Him and confessing our faith."[52]

Having argued that the proper end of *religio* is God, Aquinas immediately confronts the obvious objection that religion cannot be *only* about God because the New Testament itself, in one of the rare biblical uses of the term "religion" (Gk. *threskeia*), adjures believers that "religion that God our Father accepts as pure and faultless is this: to look after orphans and widows and to keep oneself from being polluted by the world"[53]—both of which involve a lot more than a believer's individual experience of God. Aquinas readily grants this objection, in a response that bears quoting in full because it has important implications for how "religion" is treated in the empirical literature:

> Religion has two kinds of acts. Some are its proper and immediate acts, which it elicits, and by which man is directed to God alone, for instance, sacrifice, adoration, and the like. But it has other acts, which it produces through the

medium of the virtues which it commands, directing them to the honor of God, because the virtue which is concerned with the end, commands the virtues which are concerned with the means. Accordingly *to visit the fatherless and widows in their tribulation* is an act of religion as commanding, and an act of mercy as eliciting; and *to keep oneself unspotted from this world* is an act of religion as commanding, but of temperance or some other virtue as eliciting.[54]

In other words, for Aquinas the scope of "religion" can be considered narrowly or broadly. Narrowly, it can be construed as specific cultic or devotional practices of which the primary end is to render a certain service to God: in this list of "proper and immediate acts" he includes devotion (*devotio*), prayer (*oratione*), adoration (*adoratio*), sacrifice (*sacrificium*), oblations (*oblationes*), tithes (*decimae*), vows (*voti*), oaths (*iurare*), adjuration (*adiurare*), and invocation (*invocatio*).[55] Such acts are directed to God as an end, though they are not sufficient in themselves to *get* to God; they must themselves be informed by the divinely infused theological virtues of faith, hope, and charity.[56] But these "proper and immediate" acts of religion are, for Aquinas, neither sufficient nor comprehensive in describing the shape of a faithful Christian life, because to be directed to God as one's end entails that all of one's life, including those parts that seem quite ordinary and mundane, is also directed toward God as its final end; the moral virtue of religion commands other acts of moral virtue. So in this broader sense, the entirety of a life ordered properly to God as its end could be fruitfully considered "religious." Aquinas did not consider religion to be something unique to Christians—as above, he draws his definition of *religio* from Cicero and though he was no champion of religious liberty, he respected and advocated tolerance for the Jewish communities of his day.[57] He would not, however, have recognized Christianity as one "religion" among many, nor would he have recognized a "religious" sphere of life that was somehow categorically distinct from the "secular," nor would he have believed that "religion" is a part of life that one can opt in or out of, or discard entirely. There were no atheists to speak of in Aquinas' time; and if there had been, one suspects that he would have wanted to analyze what sort of final end such persons were acting for—and, in that, he would have recognized his or her god.

What lessons might Aquinas' thought bear for contemporary empirical work on "religion, spirituality, and health"? Again, as with "health," Aquinas would likely want researchers, clinicians, and others who talk about "religion" to consider carefully whether they mean "religion" in a narrow sense, as a set of devotional/cultic practices, or "religion" in its broader sense, as the entirety of human life oriented to God and to the worship of God. If the former, Aquinas' thought would pose no objection to the empirical investigation of the effects of these practices on bodily health (*sanitas*); though as above, he might wonder why anyone would care so deeply about the question, since the end to which religion is directed (God) is so much more important than *sanitas.* But if "religion" is invoked in this narrow sense, Aquinas would rightly caution that this not lead to a myopic vision in which "religion" is pigeonholed into a few specified devotional practices and the rest of life is considered somehow to be unrelated to these practices. Such a myopic view of cultic practices could, that is, render the broader and immensely important effects of religion—its ability to direct the other moral virtues toward the things of God—invisible, and so paradoxically diminish "religion" in an effort to highlight it. But if "religion" is understood in the broader sense, as the whole of human life directed to God and to God's things, then it is worth considering (as we will below) how empirical work on "religion and health" differs from other ways of considering what constitutes a good life, such as the modern movement of "positive psychology."

So much, then, for "religion"—but what about "spirituality"? In some ways, it would seem that "spirituality" is a concept with which Aquinas would be comfortably familiar, and of which he would make considerable use. As the prayer at the epigraph of this chapter makes clear, Aquinas was a friar and priest of considerable piety and religious feeling, so much that one of his contemporary biographers speaks of him as a "spiritual master" and devotes a volume to this aspect of his person and his work.[58] He was a great admirer and disciple of the Eastern Christian apophatic tradition, which emphasized the otherness of God and the failure of ordinary human superlatives (such as "good" or "wise") to capture God in God's essence; such words can apply to God not univocally, but only analogically.[59] Furthermore, as we have already considered above, Aquinas depicts the human as a restless wanderer, wounded by original sin and separated from the God who is the one in whom true delight can be found, yet constantly and inexorably searching for that God, aware that the pleasures of the world cannot fully and ultimately satisfy. Finding God requires not only habituation in virtue but also the gifts of the Holy Spirit that allow humans to be moved by the Spirit on the journey toward God.[60] The journey toward God involves the reception of a divinely infused created light through which the person is made "deiform";[61] and insofar as God is Spirit, this is a spiritual journey. So in many senses of the words "spirit" and "spiritual"—the Spirit of God, the spirituality of the incorporeal intellectual faculty, the spiritual gifts that equip humans for the journey to God—Aquinas would both recognize and embrace "spirituality" as a welcome and necessary facet of human life.

What Aquinas would not recognize, and which would be entirely alien to his thought, is any account of "spirituality" that divorced it from "religion," as if one could have the former without the latter. We may recall that for Aquinas the works of the moral virtue of *religio* included the "interior acts" of devotion and prayer, such that these practices are an essential component of the religious life.[62] Acts such as these are clearly situated in the structure of a life oriented toward God as its final end, and are accountable to a tradition for their formation and regulation. If an individual were to practice these interior acts but to neglect the public performance of the exterior acts of *religio* such as adoration and tithing (not to mention, for example, the reception of the sacraments), Aquinas would hold that such a person was manifesting a truncated and inadequate habituation into *religio.* But if an individual were to abandon the explicit referent of a particular god altogether and to proclaim him- or herself "spiritual, but not religious," in the sense that he or she wanted to have transcendence and beauty without the encumbrance of "organized religion," Aquinas would see a person searching for beatitude and yet, tragically, lacking the light to find it. Insofar as "spirituality" in modern culture names a lack of teleological openness in modern life, Aquinas would regard it as a hopeful, if incomplete, sign that might prompt humans to more fruitful searching. But insofar as "spirituality" is taken as a possible end in itself, as a more flexible alternative to "religion," Aquinas would regard it as a presumptuous desire to attain a semblance of beatitude without submitting oneself to the communal discipline necessary to attain it.[63] Thomas might also look at the various attitudes and dispositions that are counted as "spiritual" in the religion, spirituality, and health literature and would wonder why certain of them (such as the ability to comfort oneself in the midst of serious illness) are counted as "spiritual" rather than, for example, simple signs of whether one is habituated in the moral virtue of courage. For all of these reasons, researchers and interpreters of the "religion, spirituality, and health" literature might do well to abolish the words "spiritual" and "spirituality" entirely from their research vocabulary; such a move would force abandonment of the false duality of "spiritual" and "religious" as well as the false duality of "spiritual" and "physical," and would force everyone to much more clear articulation of what they really believe.

THE POSSIBILITIES AND PERILS OF A (CHRISTIAN) PSYCHOLOGY OF HUMAN FLOURISHING

So far in this chapter, after reviewing some of what is wrong with particular modern interpretations of "religion," "spirituality," and "health," I have briefly and schematically described St. Thomas Aquinas' approach to the empirical sciences, to bodily health (*sanitas*) and happiness (*beatitudo*), and to religion (*religio*) and spirituality, considering what lessons Aquinas' treatment of these topics might bear for the construction and interpretation of contemporary empirical investigations in religion, spirituality, and health. I argued that such investigations might proceed with more conceptual clarity (and more faithfully to the Christian theological tradition) if more careful attention is given to exactly what is intended by "religion" and "health." "Spirituality," however, is a problematic concept in its modern usage when opposed to "religion": Aquinas, I argued, understood spiritual practice only in the context of a life oriented toward the things of God. Such spirituality is not opposed to religion, but integral to it. For that reason, I argued, "spirituality" could be fruitfully abolished, forcing those who use the term, by using other modes of description, to be more clear in what they intend by it.

This chapter so far has primarily been a critical one, with much more to say about what is wrong with the modern "religion, spirituality, and health" movement than about what a plausible Thomistic modification of it might be. It is indeed often easier and safer to be critical than it is to be constructive; but such an approach would be hardly faithful to the spirit of Aquinas, who engaged in careful and charitable critique of opposing views only that he might then offer a constructive distinction or account that might retain what was good in them and jettison what was wrong. In this spirit, therefore, it seems right to conclude with a schematic proposal for what an empirical research program in "religion and health" might look like, if informed by Thomistic principles.

First, such a movement would understand its use of empirical method not as an attempt to "explain away" religious belief and practice, nor as an attempt to harness it for instrumental and/or consumer-driven ends, but as a way to learn more about the biological, psychological, and social configurations of wayfarers on their way to God. Insofar as "religion" is an embodied habit that entails bodily practices, the methods of the empirical sciences may fruitfully be applied to it. But insofar as the empirical sciences cannot exhaustively comprehend the essence of the human person, who exists not as body alone but as a body-soul unity with a divinely given openness to the incorporeal, so also the empirical sciences cannot exhaustively comprehend "religion" or, for that matter, any other aspect of the human moral life. The empirical sciences can therefore take an honored and important place, which also happens to be a limited and humble place, within the analysis of human life and human action.

Second, because "health" so often fills the same sort of teleological role in our day that *beatitudo* filled in the work of Aquinas, and because *religio,* in its broadest sense, encompasses much more than its specific and proper devotional acts, a Thomistically informed "religion and health" movement would understand itself, most broadly, as a science of human flourishing. Such a movement would want to know what sorts of bodily and psychological configurations reflect and/or contribute to flourishing, and what sorts of these configurations detract from it. In this, of course, it would have obvious parallels with a nascent discipline even younger than the "religion, spirituality, and health" movement, that of "positive psychology."[64] Like "positive psychology," a Thomistic empirical investigation of human psychology would want to discern not only how humans languish and suffer, but also how they flourish, and would want to learn more about the biopsychosocial contexts and configurations that might provide the most favorable conditions for that flourishing. Also like "positive psychology," it would want to further specify what the virtues look like in a twenty-first-century context (as opposed to Aquinas' thirteenth-century context) and would want to know how such virtues and habits are acquired and lost. It is no accident, in this regard, that some modern psychological scholars informed by the work of Aquinas have warmly welcomed "positive psychology" as an advance within the field of psychology as a whole.[65]

There is, however, at least one significant difference between the sort of Thomistically informed science of flourishing which I am proposing and "positive psychology" as it is currently shaped, a difference that has to do with the ends envisioned by each of these fields. Human flourishing, in either an Aristotelian or Thomistic sense, is not self-interpreting, nor is its discernment a matter of individualistic, subjective judgment about the state of one's own life. Human flourishing, rather, is discerned by those who are sufficiently habituated in virtue so as to have the eyes to recognize flourishing where it appears. Correlatively, the "virtues" also are not self-interpreting. Virtues, for both Aristotle and

Aquinas, take their form in response to the needs of a particular *polis* or *civitas*: those habits that when embodied contribute to the flourishing of the *civitas* are therefore virtuous. It is useful, therefore, to consider what sort of *civitas* is sustained by the virtues of the positive psychology movement, which Peterson and Seligman[66] classify generically as "wisdom and knowledge," "courage," "humanity," "justice," "temperance," and "transcendence," the latter of which comprises such subvirtues as "appreciation of beauty and excellence," "gratitude," "hope," "humor," and "spirituality." What is notable about Peterson and Seligman's list is that their virtues are intelligible with an immanent, this-worldly frame of reference, and although they beckon toward the "transcendent," they require no articulation or commitment as to what the nature of the "transcendent" is. There is no space within the taxonomy, for example, for what Aquinas called "theological virtues," habits that are unintelligible within an imminent frame, which require supernatural infusion, and which require the existence of a loving God to maintain. Peterson and Seligman's virtues, in other words, turn out to correlate quite well to the needs of a modern, liberal social order in which individuals are bound by a desire for peaceful and minimally intrusive coexistence without any commitment to the articulation of shared ends.

A Thomistic science of flourishing would applaud the whole of Peterson and Seligman's work, but it would refuse to bind itself or its articulation of the virtues to the moral minimalism of the liberal social order. As stated above, the *civitas* toward which Aquinas' virtues are correlative is the Augustinian *civitas Dei,* the communion of the saints defined by and unified in its love for God and God's eternal *ratio.* Such a revised conception of the *civitas* toward which virtues are correlative not only invites "transcendence" but, for its fulfillment, requires it: human flourishing is ultimately realized only in the active, doxological rest of the beatific vision of God. Virtues are only true virtues, and "health" only true health, if they lead to, or at least do not hinder, the pursuit of *this* end. A fully Thomistic empirical science of human flourishing would, therefore, robustly own its ends and name its *civitas.* Such an account clearly requires a great deal of confessional specificity, a willingness to commit to the particular claims of the Christian tradition in all (or nearly all) of the detail with which Aquinas presents them in the voluminous *Summa theologiae.*

This sort of theocentric Thomistic science of human flourishing will never be actualized outside of a robustly confessional research context (if even there), as it challenges the teleological pluralism that grants the empirical sciences much of their social legitimacy and as it would make it difficult for persons of different religious/confessional traditions (including different Christian traditions) to work together on common areas of concern. This situation calls not for despair, but for realism. Thomistic virtue theory, always celebratory of the goodness of creation and of the ability of human reason, even apart from the state of grace, to arrive at *some* truth *some* of the time[67] and to attain virtues that, though not ultimately fulfilling, are nonetheless real and good virtues,[68] provides plenty of space for good-willed persons of different moral and religious tradition to look for areas of common agreement, to celebrate those agreements, and collaboratively to pursue shared efforts. But the very real political need for adherents of different religious persuasions to join collaboratively in research efforts and to present the results and interpretations of such research to a pluralistic, liberally formed audience, however necessary and justified, holds the "religion, spirituality, and health" movement hostage in what can only be described as a tragic situation. Specifically, the politically mandated abstraction of research programs from confessionally specific ends forces research in "religion, spirituality, and health" to deprive itself of the teleological and theological contexts within which most religious traditions, including Christianity, derive their life-giving power. It should be no surprise, then, that theologically minded interpreters often find research in "religion, spirituality, and health" to be somewhat general and anemic: such generality is the price of legitimacy within the modern, liberal culture of the psychological and medical sciences.

To modern researchers, clinicians, and interpreters of the contemporary literature of "religion, spirituality, and health" who are not yet willing to countenance the sort of teleological particular research program that I am gesturing toward here, the thought of St. Thomas can still provide a helpful and possibly life-giving context. At the very least, Thomistic thought invites and forces those who engage it to consider and articulate the operative final cause(s) toward which all of their actions are directed as an end. It teaches that human life is not static, that on every level it has a directedness, that it is *going* somewhere or moving *toward* (or away from) something; and so it forces interpreters to attune themselves to the contexts within which human action becomes intelligible. And above all, it reminds readers that "religion" and perhaps "spirituality," as particular instances of human experience and action, are also not static, but exist in a robustly particular context. This robustly particular context, in Aquinas' narrative, entails an ineffable and incomprehensible God who yet became human to draw humans into an eternal life of light and beauty in which all desires find their fulfillment. Commonly used words like "spirituality," "transcendence," and even "ecstasy" do not even approximate the intensity of this beauty; indeed, no words do. But for Aquinas, who appreciated both the power and the limitation of human language, that is just the way that things should be.

NOTES

1. From Thomas Aquinas, "Longer Prayer After Communion," *The Aquinas Prayer Book: The Prayers and Hymns of St. Thomas Aquinas*, trans. and ed. Robert Anderson and Johann Moser (Manchester, NH: Sophia Institute Press, 2000), 82–85.
2. See, for example, Larry Culliford, *The Psychology of Spirituality: An Introduction* (London: Jessica Kingsley Publishers, 2011).
3. Robert Wuthnow, *After Heaven: Spirituality in America Since the 1950s* (Berkeley: University of California Press, 1998).
4. Jeremy Carrette and Richard King, *Selling Spirituality: The Silent Takeover of Religion* (New York: Routledge, 2005).
5. Jacqueline S. Mattis, "African American Women's Definitions of Spirituality and Religiosity," *Journal of Black Psychology* 26 (2000): 101–22; Lisa M. Lewis, Sheila Henkin, Diane Reynolds, and Bengal Ogedegbe, "African American Spirituality: A Process of Honoring God, Others, and Self," *Journal of Holistic Nursing* 25 (2007): 6–23.

6. Yuk-Lin Renita Wong and Jana Vinsky, "Speaking from the Margins: A Critical Reflection on the 'Spiritual-but-not-Religious' Discourse in Social Work," *British Journal of Social Work* 39 (2009): 1343–59.
7. Nicholas Lash, *The Beginning and the End of 'Religion'* (New York: Cambridge University Press, 1996), 12.
8. Joel James Shuman and Keith G. Meador, *Heal Thyself: Spirituality, Medicine, and the Distortion of Christianity* (New York: Oxford University Press, 2003), 6.
9. Ibid., 74.
10. Ibid., 6.
11. Arthur L. Caplan, H. Tristram Engelhardt Jr., and James J. McCartney, eds., *Concepts of Health and Disease: Interdisciplinary Perspectives* (Reading, MA: Addison-Wesley, 1981).
12. Harold G. Koenig and David B. Larson, "Use of Hospital Services, Religious Attendance, and Religious Affiliation," *Southern Medical Journal* 91 (1998): 925–32.
13. Kenneth I. Pargament, Bruce W. Smith, Harold G. Koenig, and Lisa Perez, "Patterns of Positive and Negative Religious Coping with Major Life Stressors," *Journal for the Scientific Study of Religion* 37 (1998): 710–24.
14. Amy H. Peterman, George Fitchett, Marianne J. Brady, Lesbia Hernandez, and David Cella, "Measuring Spiritual Well-Being in People With Cancer: The Functional Assessment of Chronic Illness Therapy—Spiritual Well-Being Scale (FACIT-Sp)," *Annals of Behavioral Medicine* 24 (2002): 49–58.
15. Michiyo Ando, Tatsuya Morita, Tatsuo Akechi, and Takuya Okamoto, "Efficacy of Short-Term Life-Review Interviews on the Spiritual Well-Being of Terminally Ill Cancer Patients," *Journal of Pain and Symptom Management* 39 (2010): 993–1002; Zora Djuric, Josephine Mirasolo, LaVern Kimbrough, Diane R. Brown, Lance K. Heilbrun, Lisa Canar, Raghu Venkatranamamoorthy, and Michael S. Simon, "A Pilot Trial of Spirituality Counseling for Weight Loss Maintenance in African American Breast Cancer Survivors," *Journal of the National Medical Association* 101 (2009): 552–64.
16. Ando et al., "Efficacy of Short-Term Life-Review Interviews on the Spiritual Well-Being of Terminally Ill Cancer Patients."
17. Shuman and Meador, *Heal Thyself*.
18. Throughout this chapter, in quoting from the *Summa theologiae,* sometimes referred to as the *Summa Theologica,* I draw from Thomas Aquinas, *Summa Theologica,* 5 vols., trans. Fathers of the English Dominican Province (Notre Dame, IN: Christian Classics, 1981). Specific references to this work in the notes will take the form (*STh* part.question.article), such that, for example, (*STh* I-II.2.1) refers to the first part of the second part (*Prima secundae*), question 2, article 1.
19. *STh* I.84.6.
20. Armand A. Maurer, *Medieval Philosophy*, 2nd ed. (Toronto: Pontifical Institute of Medieval Studies, 1982), 154.

21. *STh* I.84.1.
22. *STh* I.84.6.
23. *STh* I-II.37.4.
24. *STh* I.1.1.*resp*.
25. Ibid.
26. *STh* I-II.6–21.
27. *STh* I-II.22–48.
28. *STh* I-II.49–54.
29. Preamble of the Constitution of the World Health Organization as adopted by the International Health Conference: 1948, New York, June 19–22, 1946; signed on July 22, 1946, by the representatives of sixty-one states (Official Records of the WHO, no. 2, p. 100) and entered into force on April 7, 1948.
30. For a provocative raising of this question, see Gerald P. McKenny, *To Relieve the Human Condition: Bioethics, Technology, and the Body* (Albany: State University of New York Press, 1997).
31. Jonathan M. Metzl and Anna Kirkland, eds., *Against Health: How Health Became the New Morality* (New York: New York University Press, 2010).
32. *STh* I-II.63.4.
33. *STh* I-II.2–3.
34. *STh* I-II.2.4.4.
35. *STh* I-II.2.5.
36. *STh* II-II.23.8.
37. *STh* I.75–89.
38. *STh* I-II.22–48.
39. *STh* I-II.49–54.
40. *STh* I-II.55–67.
41. *STh* I-II.63.3.
42. *STh* I-II.65.2.
43. *STh* I-II.38.5.
44. *STh* I-II.73.3.
45. *STh* I.13.5.
46. *STh* I-II.49.1.
47. *STh* I-II.49.3.
48. Eleonore Stump, *Aquinas* (New York: Routledge, 2003), 37.
49. *STh* I.84.7–8.
50. Andrew Newberg, Eugene D'Aquili, and Vince Rouse, *Why God Won't Go Away: Brain Science and the Biology of Belief* (New York: Ballantine, 2002).
51. *STh* II-II.80.1.
52. *STh* II-II.81.1.*resp*.
53. James 1:27 (NIV).
54. *STh* II-II.81.1.*ad1*.
55. *STh* II-II.82–91.
56. *STh* II-II.81.5.
57. *STh* II-II.10.11.
58. Jean-Pierre Torrell, *Saint Thomas Aquinas, Vol 2.: Spiritual Master*, trans. Robert Royal (Washington, DC: Catholic University of America Press, 2003).
59. *STh* I.13.2, 5.
60. *STh* I-II.68.1–2.
61. *STh* I.12.5.
62. *STh* II-II.82–83.
63. cf. *STh* II-II.21.
64. Christopher Peterson and Martin E. P. Seligman, *Character Strengths and Virtues: A Handbook and Classification* (New York: Oxford University Press, 2004).
65. Paul C. Vitz, "Psychology in Recovery," *First Things* (March 2005): 17–21.
66. Peterson and Seligman, *Character Strengths and Virtues*.
67. *STh* I.1.1.
68. *STh* I-II.63.4.

M. THERESE LYSAUGHT

7. BEGUILING RELIGION

The Bifurcations and Biopolitics of Spirituality and Medicine[1]

In an article entitled "Meeting My Mother Again," John Carmody, once an ordained Catholic priest but now twenty years estranged from the church, chronicles his experience of dying of cancer. As he lay in his hospital bed, a priest appears and asks if he wishes to be anointed. "With no thought," he says "yes." The sacrament surprises him. "It began almost shamefully casually," he admits, yet it proved to be, in his words, "the most moving moment in my month's stay in the hospital." "Indeed" he notes, it "lodged itself among the half-dozen most moving religious experiences in my life."[2] This from what he describes as "a spare, adapted version of the church's ancient ritual" and "at most ten minutes of unpretentious prayer."

From the perspective of patients and families, anointing of the sick is a powerful religious practice. Again and again, Carmody's experience is echoed in the corridors of medicine. Every day in the twenty-first-century United States, this scenario is repeated—in hospitals, in hospices, sometimes in parishes, sometimes in homes. Christians faced with serious or mortal illness summon their pastor or a priest on staff, and sometimes surrounded by family and friends, sometimes accompanied by health care professionals, they are prayed over, prayed with, and allow oil to be applied to their foreheads, their hands, other bodily sites of pain.

In my own life, anointing has surfaced in unexpected places. My own children, born eight weeks early, were anointed on their second day of life by a Catholic priest in a Seventh-Day Adventist hospital. I have been particularly struck and moved by the stories of three of my friends, three (academic) women, who are each equally ambiguous about the church. On separate occasions each of these friends have testified to me—unprompted and unaware of the centrality of anointing to my research agenda—of how strikingly powerful their own participation in the sacrament of anointing proved to be as each sat by the side of her dying mother. For each, anointing proved to be deeply moving in ways they could scarcely articulate.

Stories and experiences like these—of the power of religious practices, especially for those experiencing illness or negotiating dying—have fueled the recent exponential growth in the scholarship and literature surrounding the relationship of spirituality, theology, health, and medicine. As a theologian, I should be encouraged by this interest and the ways that it might renew the long-standing relationship between faith and medicine, a relationship that flourished for 1,500 years in the West but with the emergence of modernity became constructed as a conflict.[3] Yet as a theologian who studies the anointing of the sick, I must confess that the field of spirituality and medicine—indeed, the biopsychosocialspiritual model as a whole—gives me great pause.[4] For this model and this newly emergent field as a whole are structured by assumptions, norms, and terminology that marginalize and relativize a practice like anointing.

On the one hand, the practice of anointing of the sick is not a "spiritual" practice—it is a "religious" practice. It remains one of the few spaces where, on a regular basis, in hospitals secular or not, religion *irrupts*—visually, tactilely, practically, publically, olfactorily—into the domain of modern medicine. When it does so, the juxtaposition between high-tech, largely effective medicine and this peculiar holdover from premodernity can be at best ambiguous or at worst jarring. Picture, if you will, the typical scenario: a priest in clerical garb enters the highly technologized space of a modern hospital room. For a brief moment, he is allowed to usurp center stage in a sea of medical personnel. He smears oil (hardly a hygienic action) on a body that is likely pumped full of pharmaceuticals, may be tethered to various forms of technology, and has perhaps only a tenuous hold on life. For that brief moment, the priest assumes authority over the space of the hospital room—the physicians and medical staff step back, perhaps uncomfortable or uncertain whether they should be present. He conducts a rite that he, as well as the patient and family, believes has the ability to heal. The philosophers' favorite conceit—the hypothetical visitor from Mars beamed into a contemporary hospital room—would no doubt perceive this performance as extraordinarily strange and out of place.[5] It is permitted, we know, if the patient wishes to have it, as a way of finding meaning or coping, but the fundamental disconnects between anointing and contemporary medicine are otherwise glossed over in silence.

One might counter that if anointing is best understood as a religious rather than a spiritual practice, then it might be better mapped not to spirituality and medicine but to the subcategory of religion and health. Yet here anointing meets an entirely different set of obstacles. For as we have seen throughout this volume, the subfield of religion and health is largely concerned about efficacy and outcomes. It asks the instrumentalist question: do religious practices (or does religious participation) have a positive or negative effect on health status and health outcomes, on a population basis? Studies seeking to correlate church attendance and overall health status or examining the efficacy of prayer on clinical outcomes are now abundant. Yet as has no doubt been discussed extensively in this volume, to conceive of religious practices in these instrumentalist terms risks deforming their richer meaning, reducing them to, in Andrew Lustig's apt phrase,[6] little more than "health technologies"—useful if they produce a clinically measurable benefit but otherwise suspect or dangerous. According to this logic, we should conduct a clinical trial of anointing of the sick. What if such a study determined that anointed patients had better outcomes—ought physicians offer it as a tool within the medical armamentarium? Or alternatively, what if the study determined that patient outcomes were worse—should Christian communities stop anointing? Ought it be banned as malpractice from clinical contexts?[7]

In short, a traditional religious practice like anointing of the sick, practiced within the Christian tradition for millennia, fits tenuously at best with the framework provided by the emerging discipline of spirituality and medicine and, in fact, highlights serious problems with the philosophical infrastructure that frames the rules for conceptualizing—and practicing—religion and spirituality in the clinical setting today. I will argue that the theoretical shape of this discourse is deeply problematic for those who take religious practices seriously for at least three reasons. First, it relies on well-deconstructed dualisms, dichotomies, or binaries—a conceptual infrastructure that has been effectively debunked by most feminist, postmodern, and other contemporary philosophers. Such dualisms, as we will see, serve to position religion such that it lies on the nonnormative side of the divide—thereby devaluing and disempowering religion *vis a vis* spirituality. Second, I will argue that the discourse on spirituality and medicine emerged when it did and in the way it did because it provided a crucial component of the consolidation of the biopolitical character of modern medicine. As we will see, thirdly, this aspect of the field of spirituality and medicine mirrors a similar trend seen in the field of bioethics. The biopsychosocialspiritual model in medicine emerged alongside the field of bioethics in the mid-to-late 1970s, both serving to effectively marginalize religion, theology, and modes of substantive rationality except where they could be transformed into instrumental modalities. In the end, I will propose that, properly understood, the practice of anointing—as well as other authentic religious practices—ought well be seen as deeply subversive of the configuration of contemporary accounts of spirituality and medicine.

BINARIES, BIFURCATIONS, DICHOTOMIES, AND DUALISMS: THE PHILOSOPHICAL POSITIONING OF RELIGION

The literature on spirituality and medicine or religion and health is structured according to now well-deconstructed dualisms, dichotomies, or binaries.[8] This is not a little ironic, insofar as the turn to the biopscyhosocialspiritual model in the 1970s was proposed as a way to overcome a number of dichotomies or binary oppositions deemed problematic in twentieth-century medicine, particularly its reductionistic materialism found in its focus on the body as a machine.[9] In the following section, I sketch four intertwined dualisms that shape the field of spirituality and medicine: (1) form versus content (or substance or matter), (2) mind versus body, (3) subjective versus objective, and (4) private versus public.[10] As with most dualistic structures, one pole of each binary is consistently privileged as normative—in this case, it is the formal, the mental, the subjective, the private that merits positive valuation. Not surprisingly, these emerge as the characteristics of "spirituality." More or less subtly, the opposite pole—that which maps content, body, objectivity, and public—is devalued, positioned, carefully delimited, and circumscribed. It is here that we find "religion," including substantively religious practices like the anointing of the sick. Although each of these binaries could be described in much greater detail and a legion of examples educed from the literature in support, allow me to briefly summarize each.

Spirituality as Formal

The distinction between form and matter (or form/content or form/substance) has a long history within the Western philosophical tradition. While the meaning of the terms and relationships between them shifted from Plato to Aristotle to Descartes to Hobbes to the logical empiricists and beyond, it is Kant's revision of the terms that continues to inform contemporary discourse. Formal entities are, for Kant, abstract, necessary, universal concepts, forms of intuition, innate in the human mind, and, importantly, independent of human experience (therefore *a priori*). They are true for everyone, everywhere regardless of content. Mathematical truths, for example, are formal: 2+2 always equals 4 independent of the things added, whether one is counting boxes, money, or human beings.

Assertions of the formal, *a priori* nature of spirituality are ubiquitous within the field of spirituality and medicine. Christina Puchalski, an internist and geriatrician who has pioneered the practice of spiritual assessment, especially in end-of-life care, succinctly captures this conviction:

> I see spirituality as that which allows a person to experience transcendent meaning in life. This is often expressed as a relationship with God, but it can also be about nature, art, music, family or community—whatever beliefs and values give a person a sense of meaning and purpose in life.[11]

Chaplain Thomas St. James O'Connor concurs, finding among his research subjects: "All believe that everyone is spiritual *whether that person recognizes it or not*, for meaning-making is an essential part of being human."[12] Or, finally, palliative care physician Tomasz R. Okon notes that for the literature on spirituality and medicine: "Regardless of one's particular spiritual orientation, every individual has to make a decision as to whether one's life has meaning and value that extends beyond self, life and death. Even a focused and resolute answer negating such meaning places one in relation to the transcendent."[13]

In other words, try as one might, one cannot escape being spiritual. This, of course, is a Kantian sort of claim, a formal claim—it holds that spirituality is a fundamental, inalienable human category, something fundamental to who we are as human persons. It holds that spirituality is a neutral, universal constituent of human being; its content doesn't matter.[14] In this way, spirituality holds a similar position to that of the faculty of autonomy in bioethics. It is this formal nature that allows "spirituality" to be assessed more or less scientifically.

One can, of course, escape being religious. Religions are clearly not universal, necessary, innate. They are particular and chosen; one is initiated into a religion through a series of rites or practices. One might convert from religion A to religion B, one's Catholicism might lapse, or one might decide to declare oneself an agnostic or atheist. Religions are, by definition and at times by proclamation, particular, defined by highly contingent histories (e.g., the Incarnation, Gautama's decision to seek Enlightenment). Religions are, if anything, defined by their content and substantive claims—their particular beliefs, practices, histories, convictions, and communities.

Thus, in casting spirituality as part of the transcendental *a priori* structure of the human person, the field of spirituality and medicine creates problems for religion. While required to respect that all persons are spiritual, health care professionals must remain skeptical or agnostic about particular religious claims and practices. But, as with all formal claims, this approach also creates problems for spirituality. As Wilfred McSherry and Keith Cash note in their 2004 comprehensive review of the taxonomy of the language of spirituality: "the term 'spirituality' as used within nursing is problematic and in danger of becoming so broad and empty that it is meaningless," and that "a universal definition of spirituality may be theoretically and culturally impossible."[15]

Spirituality as a Mental Construct

Advocates of spirituality in medicine often champion the new attention to spirituality as a way of overcoming the problematic dualism of mind versus body so often encountered in medicine, a rupture often attributed to the work of Rene Descartes. As Puchalski notes: "More physicians are becoming aware of the unity of the human person—that is, body and spirit—and therefore are integrating spiritual care into their practice of medicine."[16]

However, the current construct of spirituality in medicine furthers this dualism. It does so in three ways. First, spirituality is cast as a categorical orientation of the human person located in the faculty of decision. Recall Okon's comment earlier:

> Regardless of one's particular spiritual orientation, every individual has to make *a decision* as to whether one's life has meaning and value that extends beyond self, life and death. Even a focused and resolute answer negating such meaning places one in relation to the transcendent.[17]

Again, the content of one's orientation or decision—the choice one actually makes—is irrelevant; one can even "negate such meaning."

What matters is that a decision, a choice is made.[18] A "decision," of course, is an activity of the reason and the will—in other words, spirituality is located as mental construct. Such a position is, once again, a good Kantian position.

Spirituality is further distanced from the body by the bifurcation of spirituality from religion or religiosity. O'Connor and associates helpfully articulate the standard distinction:

> Spirituality is viewed as distinct from religiosity. Religiosity is an expression of faith through the practices of a particular religion or denomination. . . . [S]pirituality as meaning-making does not necessarily have to be expressed in a religious or denominational context.[19]

Thus, one might be spiritual but not religious (believing in a higher being without religious affiliation or practices), religious but not spiritual (participating in external religious practices without conscious commitment to meaning-making), or both spiritual and religious.[20] Here the term "spiritual" pertains primarily to "meaning" or sometimes is expanded to include "beliefs"—both of which are, again, mental constructs—while the term "religious" is typically applied to the external social, cultural, and/or institutional aspects of transcendent concerns, to the rituals, devotions, or practices of a tradition—in other words, to those things that people do with their bodies.

Thus in all of these configurations, spirituality remains a mental construct abstracted by definition from practices, embodiment, community, formation, and more.[21] Mind-body dualism has not been overcome, but is in fact reinforced.

Spirituality as Subjective

The subjective-objective dichotomy operates in the field of spirituality and medicine in two ways. First, it structures the discourse itself. The very framing of the question—spirituality and medicine—is predicated on this polarity. It presupposes that spirituality and medicine are two different realms that somehow must be connected. Medicine, via the empirical method and biological reductionism, firmly staked its claim to the mantle of objectivity throughout the twentieth century. As a mental construct, spirituality cannot but be firmly lodged in individual subjectivity, while medicine and science map without remainder the objective side of the Cartesian divide. Pastoral counselor Gary Shogren notes: "[Even] in an age when medical technology has taken on religious connotations of its own . . . religion and science [remain] neatly divided into Cartesian categories, with healing generally falling into the realm of science."[22] Moreover, the turn to spirituality in medicine in the 1970s and 1980s was and remains part of a broader series of initiatives intentionally designed to integrate patients' subjective experiences, feelings, and values into the clinical context. Spirituality, as illustrative questions from a variety of spiritual assessment instruments indicates, concerns subjective experiences and feelings: "How close do you feel to God?"; "A reason I pray by myself is because I enjoy praying"; "I feel thankful for my blessings"; and so forth.[23]

This distinction that places religion/spirituality in the space of subjectivity and science/medicine in objectivity relies on and reinforces particular epistemological assumptions ubiquitous in this literature, namely, that science and medicine make *truth* claims, while the same cannot be said about spirituality or religion. At best, advocates will affirm that spirituality provides individuals with "their own" truth, but this truth follows decidedly different epistemological rules; it is, if it exists, more "mystical" and therefore about it we must be apophatic.[24] Here the objective pole is—at least momentarily—privileged with regard to truth, but the subjective pole is privileged with regard to meaning.

At the same time, however, the subject-object polarity also structures the relationship between spirituality and religion. Spirituality continues to occupy the subjective pole, while religion becomes associated with the objective. Being linked to the objective, however, does not award religion with the status of truth that is conferred to medicine (although religion is often critiqued for making unwarranted truth claims). Instead, subjectively construed spirituality becomes privileged *vis a vis* meaning and truth insofar as spirituality itself represents a truth about the human condition. Spiritual practices, feelings, and experiences chosen by patients assume a sort of noumenal unassailability. Religion, on the other hand, in its messy contingency and particularity and reliance on revelation (at least in part), becomes increasingly surd. It remains tolerated as a present yet accidental feature of many patients' lives, yet one senses in the literature an undercurrent of impatience. This predisposition makes itself clearest in allied contexts, for example, in bioethics where it is religion, especially objective teachings of religious authorities—not spirituality—that creates so many of the "dilemmas" in bioethics.[25] As Daniel Hall, Harold Koenig, and Keith Meador note in their article "Conceptualizing 'Religion': How Language Shapes and Constrains Knowledge in the Study of Religion and Health":

> In oversimplified terms, the Enlightenment paradigm approaches religion as a sort of "frosting" that may or may not be applied to the "vanilla cake" of generic human experience (Wolterstorff 2001a, 7). The frosting may come in several different flavors (Christian, Buddhist, Muslim), but the vanilla cake remains the same from person to person. In fact, the frosting is even optional to the extent that an atheist may choose to enjoy the cake without any frosting at all. Religion is thus perceived as a type of knowledge that may be added to the foundation built by reason and empiricism—but because it is not universal, religion is considered both optional and less trustworthy than the foundational knowledge shared by all humans and verified by our common sensory experience.[26]

Hall and associates testify to the ongoing struggle regarding the truth-claims religion seeks to make as a source of knowledge. Thus, while placed on the scientific side of the subjective-objective divide, religious epistemology is insufficiently empirical to prove a trustworthy source of knowledge. Equally, spirituality's nature as a foundational human intuition shared by all humans renders it more trustworthy than religion. Too savvy, however, to pretend to compete head-to-head with an empirical scientific epistemology, those who promote spirituality in medicine direct its purview away from knowledge toward the domains of "meaning" and "coping."[27] As we will see, the field of spirituality and medicine attempts to compensate for this self-avowed subjectivity by adopting the quasi-empirical tool of spiritual assessment or the more rigorous double-blind clinical trials. Not surprisingly, the methodologies and validity of many such studies are being called into question.

Spirituality as Radically, Individually Private

A category that is both mentalist and subjective cannot be other than private and radically individual. As O'Connor and colleagues hold:

> Each person makes sense of his or her life. . . . [S]pirituality [thus] is private and involves judgment. The meaning of one's life, the meaning of one's relationship with self, others and God, and the meaning one attaches to experience and events are personal and often private.[28]

Intriguingly, while O'Connor's ethnographic research found support for this perspective among patients, an agnostic amongst their cohort challenged this presupposition: "One patient, who is an agnostic, enjoyed talking about issues concerning life's meaning. He invited the researcher to debate with him the existence of God. Spirituality for him was a public matter, not a private one."[29] Again, as with the assertion that all persons are spiritual, the data confound the assumptions.

The claim that spirituality is private and individual makes possible the position that assessing and addressing patient spirituality is essential for enhancing patient autonomy. Yet here again we meet another irony, insofar as spiritual claims are inherently heteronomous. In "relating themselves to the transcendent" (whatever it is) individuals by definition cede or at least acknowledge the power that transcendent holds over their lives.

It is this heteronomy that is captured in the root of the term "religion"—*re-ligio*—re-ligate, to tie together. Religion claims to be that which again connects human persons with the transcendent.[30] Unlike the heteronomy of spirituality, this heteronomy is not personal or private but public. From the earliest uses of the term (eighth to twelfth centuries), the term "religion" meant a "state of life bound by religious vows; the condition of belonging to a religious order."[31] Religion was a public way of life embarked upon by public professions. Over time, the term broadened to encompass human "action or conduct" based on this connection to the transcendent, be they the public action of religious rituals or public adherence to a code of living in everyday life.

Thus, in the field of spirituality and medicine, where spirituality is fashioned as formal, mental, subjective, and radically individualistic and private, religion constructed is substantive, embodied, objective, and inescapably communal and public. Religion makes truth-claims and engages ensouled bodies through visible, external, communal public practices—just like its counterpart medicine. Although once inextricably intertwined and necessarily subordinated to significant and enduring religious practices, the kernel of spirituality has now been freed from the prison-house husk of religion. As such, it poses no threat to the hegemony of medicine within the clinical setting. What is more, by tranquilizing religion, spirituality and medicine allows medicine to expand its jurisdiction unimpeded. For that account, let us turn to the next section.

BEHIND BINARIES AND BIFURCATIONS: SPIRITUALITY AND MEDICINE AS BIOPOLITICS

Constructed, confined, circumscribed . . . *packaged* by these philosophical dualisms, religion is bifurcated from spirituality and marginalized or at least very carefully positioned *vis a vis* the clinical setting. One could ascribe this positioning of religion as simply the outcome of the unsophisticated adoption of modernist philosophical habits. Yet those acquainted with a hermeneutics of suspicion must always ask: whose interest does such a positioning serve? Is there more to this history? How did such a bifurcation come to be created? Moreover, as noted in this book's prologue, the field of spirituality and medicine has grown exponentially over the past three decades, in part fueled by funding from the National Institutes of Health. One can think about the history of the field and ask why did it appear when it did? How did the field of medicine—having narrated its identity over against religion for the better part of two centuries—come to so blithely accept the incorporation of spirituality-as-a-science into its domain? How did a government putatively committed to a separation between religion and state come to fund research on spirituality and health?

In this section, I will sketch initial answers to these questions by turning to Max Weber and Michel Foucault. Informed by a more sociocritical perspective on this new field of spirituality and medicine, one might argue that spirituality has been allowed to enter the realm of contemporary medicine in this new way for one simple reason: packaged in this particular philosophical configuration, it enhances the scope and power of medicine and solidifies medicine's ability to further the ends of the social order. The field of spirituality and medicine functions, in other words, as a disciplinary mode of modern, scientific "biopolitics," serving to reproduce, in and through individual bodies, the ideological commitments of contemporary culture.[32] Moreover, this new field of spirituality and medicine parallels the trajectory of another discipline that explosively came-to-be during the same time period: bioethics. Elsewhere, I have argued that bioethics has become a mode of biopolitics.[33] Not surprisingly, we find striking parallels in the fortunes of religion within both fields.

Allow me to begin with a brief overview of the notion of biopolitics, indicating as we go the various ways in which the field of spirituality and medicine interfaces with a biopolitical framework. Biopolitics, for Foucault, names an integrated set of strategies for policing and controlling populations, for "increasingly ordering all realms under the guise of improving the welfare of the individual and the population" but whose real and masked purpose is to reproduce and further the dominant social order.[34] For Foucault, a vital constituent of biopolitics from the end of the eighteenth century forward was biomedicine.[35]

To see the contemporary conversation on spirituality and medicine as a mode of biopolitics is to suggest that behind the rhetoric of freedom, empowerment, meaning, and improving the welfare of individual patients and the health of the population overall, the contemporary turn to spirituality in medicine may not actually advance patients' interests as much as it functions to shape, direct, and manage the bodies of real, human persons toward larger and perhaps hidden institutional ends.[36] How might this work?[37]

Foucault and others identify three necessary elements in biopolitical governmentality: discourses, practices, and institutions—elements we can clearly trace in the conversation on spirituality and medicine. Discourses are bodies of concepts, literatures, that define and produce objects of knowledge, that govern the ways a topic can be meaningfully talked about, reasoned about, studied. They are, in other words, academic, scholarly, professional fields. The formation of new discourses generally entails a discontinuous trajectory—careful historical work will plot the emergence of a new discourse out of the decline of an old one. Such histories will be those of ruptures, radical breaks, and useful contingencies. However, those who tell the story of the new discipline—history is generally written by the winners—will recount its emergence as a seamless, natural, logical, necessary next step in progress toward truth.

The discourse on spirituality and medicine was catalyzed in the late 1970s with George Engel's development of the biopsychosocial model for medicine.[38] For Engel and others, the biopsychosocial model of medicine arose in response to deficiencies in the functional biological/physiological approach of an increasingly technologized medicine that reached a particular apex (or nadir, depending on one's viewpoint) in the late 1960s and early 1970s. The dogmatic biological reductionism of this "biomedical model" fails to account, Engel argues, for nonphysical dimensions of human illness, healing, and patient experiences, excludes nonphysical disorders from medicine, and fails to recognize its own cultural constructedness.[39] The newly proposed biopsychosocial model (later expanded to the biopsychosocialspiritual model) provides a way to address all these dimensions of the crisis, naturally emerging as a necessary and logical development in the progress of modern medicine. Engel's seminal article launched a movement that followed the typical discursive path—the exponential development of journals, conferences, a professional literature, college classes, centers, and various graduate degrees over the course of the next two decades. As with all processes of discursive formation, the knowledge produced within this field becomes increasingly technical, formal, and esoteric, necessarily the purview of specialists and elite professionals. Consequently, as in all discursive formation, we find the creation of new health care professionals—in this case, chaplains, spiritual care, or pastoral care providers—those who have the necessary expertise to research and deploy the esoteric findings of this new field. Spirituality as a scientific discipline is no longer accessible by mere mortals, or even physicians, no matter how personal, subjective, universal, and private spirituality is claimed to be.

Discourses, of course, do not simply float free. In order to organize and discipline bodies, they must be incarnated in social *practices*, in what Foucault refers to as "techniques of discipline." Discourses and practices stand in reciprocal relationship: discourses define the rules for practices, which in turn enact those discourses *vis a vis* individual bodies.[40] Through the creation of such bodies that then go on to act in the world in self-motivated ways, practices further realize (make real) and reproduce the vision and commitments of the discourses in the world.[41]

In addition to the "dividing practice" that we have already seen—the dichotomization of religiosity and spirituality—two central practices or techniques of discipline for the field of spirituality and medicine are the now manifold instruments for spiritual assessment and the practice of taking a spiritual history.[42] Three dimensions of these practices are key to this account. First, the practice of spiritual assessment—at least as it very quickly became to be practiced within the biopsychosocial-spiritual model—is the heir of one of two contributors to medicine-as-biopolitics identified by Foucault, namely, statistical medicine or the numerical method. Physician-philosopher Jeffrey Bishop, in his important book *The Anticipatory Corpse: Medicine, Power, and the Care of the Dying*, provides a helpful account of the role of statistical medicine in the consolidation of medicine's power in the nineteenth and early twentieth centuries, particularly in areas of public health, eugenics/genetics, psychology, and sociology.[43] More importantly, he carefully demonstrates how the putatively numerical and statistical practice of spirituality scales and instruments becomes the "scientific" method of choice within this new model. As he notes, in the late 1970s "we find an explosion of new techniques to assess scientifically everything from grief to spirituality."[44] He cites a company called Psychological Assessment Resources that offers 428 different assessment tools, forty-nine of which are located under the heading "Behavior/Health." And this is but one of a myriad of such companies. The number of spiritual assessment instruments are now legion.

Second, often structured according to Likert Scales, such assessment vehicles are shaped according to the assumptions contained in the discourse on spirituality and medicine. The four-question FICA tool, for example, speaks of spirituality, faith, and beliefs rather than religion ("Do you consider yourself spiritual?") and defines the role of spirituality as meaning or comfort ("What things do you believe in that give meaning to life?"; "Does [your faith center] provide support/comfort for you during times of stress?").[45] Other approaches conceive spirituality in terms of developmental psychological functioning, *a la* Fowler's Stages of Faith[46] or as a method of psychological coping, an assumption captured in the telling acronym of one of the most commonly cited assessments developed by two of the leading figures in the spirituality and medicine field, Ken Pargament and Harold Koenig, the RCOPE.[47]

This limited psychosocial account of religion and spirituality would be less troublesome but for one key biopolitical dimension of these assessment instruments: they not only are shaped by certain assumptions about religion and spirituality, but also seek to reproduce these assumptions through the participative shaping of patients. For example, insofar as spiritual assessment instruments frame questions in terms of feelings, social support, or coping rather than terms of facts or truth, they subtly yet effectively may shape the way patients subsequently understand the nature and relevance of their own religiosity. Equally, patients who do not fit the mold may be subtly (or perhaps not so subtly) prodded in a particular direction. For example, nurse Carrie Dameron, in providing a succinct account of the very succinct

FICA assessment tool, recounts the story of one Mrs. Garcia. When asked about her spiritual beliefs, Mrs. Garcia responds: "I don't really have any spiritual beliefs or religion, but I like to go to the woods and sit quietly, listening to nature. Sometimes I take a meditation book and think about the words and sayings." Dameron interprets this finding in, *prima facie*, a peculiar manner:

> Using the FICA spiritual assessment, we discovered that Ms. Garcia says she is not spiritual, yet she practices spirituality in her life. We see that she has spiritual support through her friend and through meditation books. Ms. Garcia's assessment reveals her spiritual needs, but also communicates that the nurse is caring and open to discussing her issues. This begins a rapport between the nurse and the patient, laying the foundation for further spiritual discussions and caring nursing interventions. Later the nurse can check with Ms. Garcia and see how she is doing, continuing to assess and develop a relationship with her. Eventually the nurse might ask permission to talk further about spiritual beliefs and offer to pray with Ms. Garcia.[48]

Earlier Dameron observed that "many words Christians equate with spirituality have a Christian connotation. Examples include: church, prayer, worship, Bible, sacraments and God. Alternate words to use are faith/spiritual community, spiritual practices, meditation or quiet time, music, spiritual literature and higher/influential power or force."[49] In both cases, spiritual assessment embodies an attempt to shape patient understandings of their own spirituality/religiosity—either by shifting their words away from substantive, particular Christian language toward a spiritualized Esperanto or by imposing upon them a spirituality of which they are in possession unawares, eventually leading to religious practice! Similarly, Pargament and colleagues understand religious coping to be positive or negative. As they note: "Although the concept of coping has a positive connotation, coping can be ineffective as well as effective. Religion also has its darker side."[50] Such a perspective on religion is not simply objective and scientific. Kyle Brothers observes astutely:

> For the purposes of RCOPE, its designers narrowed the meaning of religion to religious coping. As psychology researchers, they view humans as discrete

individuals who function either successfully or unsuccessfully within society; it is because of this perspective that Pargament et al. are able to make normative claims that some religious coping is positive and some is negative. For these authors, then, the question is not only how religious coping functions in the lives of people undergoing life stressors, but also how religious coping helps or hinders functioning in society.[51]

In this way, discursive practices seek to take "unruly" bodies—bodies like those of Mrs. Garcia, of the agnostic cited earlier who believed spirituality to be public, or the 25 percent of respondents who classified themselves as neither spiritual nor religious, or those with negative religious coping—and change them, to fit them into the conceptual commitments of the new orthodoxy, thereby rendering them "docile"—amenable to the norms of medicine and the state.[52]

Finally, discursive practices are assisted in this process largely by being embedded in *institutions*, centralized social spaces that provide a visible social sanction for the claims put forward in a particular discourse. Such institutionalization is necessary for two reasons. On the one hand, it provides a place with authoritative sanction for the surveillance that is crucial for the mapping and normalizing of the bodies within a given population. On the other, as noted above, institutionally sanctioned discourses define the "normal," and through techniques and practices, they encourage individuals to regulate and achieve their own conformity with these established norms.[53] Over time, institutionalized discursive practices subtly move individuals to adopt certain attitudes and practices (e.g., that spirituality and religion are two different things) and in this way, they come to be embodied and enacted within the larger culture, prevailing as normal and acceptable. In other words, institutionalization has the effect of rendering particular discourses "true." This "truth" is reinforced via the ability of institutionalized discursive practices to "predict" normalizing outcomes and to produce "normal" bodies (to shift persons from one set of norms to another), a dance that reinforces the "scientific" character of the discourse's growing body of knowledge.

All these dimensions are captured within the field of spirituality and medicine. While resistance from clinicians continues, spirituality-as-assessable has clearly become embedded to a significant degree within the institutions of medicine and the hospital. Spiritual care professionals visit patients, they administer spiritual assessments—both now a standard part of the surveillance mechanism of modern medicine as well as a method for teaching patients certain normative concepts. Not surprisingly, the outcomes of assessment after assessment demonstrate the validity of the assessments' presuppositions (e.g., that spirituality is a universal component of the human psyche), particularly if administered to radically different demographic populations. The results of these assessments enable practitioners to intervene with patients, to normalize those unruly who might prove disruptive to the smooth flow of the medical regime. With the institutional backing of statistical science and clinical medicine, the findings from spiritual assessments are trumpeted as true, a truth reinforced by NIH funding and now thousands of studies published in prestigious sounding academic journals, backed by a plethora of "data."

As such, as Bishop rightly notes, it is not only the case that the biopsychosocialspiritual model proposed by Engel provided a solution to a crisis of biological reductionism. More significantly, Engel laid the groundwork for medicine to become totalizing. With the development of the biopsychosocialspiritual model:

> We see the deployment of the statistical sciences—particularly in psychology and social work—and the expansion of techniques of assessment to capture every dimension of human thriving. A biopsychosocialspiritual medicine is born—a medicine that addresses all features of human thriving. It sets out to nominally define, to operationally assess, and to statistically measure the wholeness of human living; it is a medicine devoted to holistic care, or perhaps better a medicine devoted to total care. Biopsychosocialspiritual medicine measures all things and is the measure of all things.[54]

From the perspective of biopower, it becomes easier to see how the discourse on spirituality and medicine was permitted to enter into and remain within the sacred space of the clinic. Rather than providing a necessary corrective to an overly reductionistic biomedicine, spirituality allied to practices of surveillance surreptitiously served to provide a way for medicine to exponentially expand the jurisdiction of its gaze and to finally marginalize the only other long-standing claimant to authority over the bodies of citizens: religion.

In this way, the story of spirituality and medicine parallels in an uncanny way the story of bioethics. Likewise launched in the mid-to-late 1970s and experiencing exponential growth as a field, the trajectory of bioethics can also be narrated as one of disciplinary formation via the development of esoteric discourses, overseen by a new profession of specialists, embodied in techniques of discipline such as informed consent, living wills, and research regulations, embedded in institutions such as laboratories, hospitals, and clinics, thereby reproducing new norms that serve not primarily the interests of the patients or physicians but rather the interests of the medical-industrial-government complex.[55]

Equally, for our purposes, this new field of bioethics—although born out of the field of theology—quickly moved to marginalize religion. By 1990, the "secularization of bioethics" was a recognized issue.[56] Kevin Wildes narrates the canonical story of the development of bioethics, maintaining that like the biopsychosocialspiritual model of medicine, bioethics emerged because of the increased technologization and biological reductionism of medicine in the 1960s. For Wildes, bioethics' initial theological character was pushed aside as a necessary, logical advance:

> [B]ioethics has emerged as a field that is distinct from theological ethics and traditional physician ethics even though both disciplines were important to the development of the field. . . . [O]ne needs to understand why theological voices receded from the field. . . . The turn toward a secular bioethics became a search for a secular or civil religion that might bind the sentiment of citizens who were at least nominally divided by religions, cultures, or other differences.[57]

Religion, in other words, is particular and divisive, unlike the universal category of spirituality, or, as those familiar with bioethics know, the main, canonical bioethics principle: autonomy.[58] The resemblances between spirituality and autonomy in these two discourses should not go unremarked. Both, of course, are formal, universal, *a priori* categories of human nature, mentalist constructions located in the rational will, contentless by definition (the content to be specified by each individual), completely subjective, and radically individual and private.[59]

Key to the marginalization of theology and religion within bioethics was a shift in modes of rationality—from substantive rationality to formal, instrumental rationality. Sociologist John H. Evans, in his book *Playing God?: Human Genetic Engineering and the Rationalization of Public Bioethical Debate*, carefully documents how the substantively rational arguments and religious language that characterized the early stages of bioethics became, by the late 1980s, systematically excluded or at least carefully positioned so as to be mostly irrelevant within public bioethics, usurped by the formal, instrumental rationality of the four principles and an emphasis on bureaucratic procedure.[60] A similar shift can be traced within the field of spirituality and medicine. As Levin suggests, early voices in this field were more interested in metaphilosophical questions (e.g., "What does this really mean?"), but these sorts of substantive questions were quickly left behind in the turn to formal modes of statistical analysis. The early pioneers in this field, as they note, were animated by "more fundamental (and one could say existential) questions about the relation of spirit and body. . . . Before the empirical research enterprise that is the contemporary religion and health field got started in earnest, about 20 years ago, theoretical discussions, especially theological discussions could be found on occasion throughout this literature."[61]

Yet Ken Vaux, Harold Vanderpool, and Paul Tillich in spirituality and medicine met the same fate as those like Paul Ramsey, Richard McCormick, and even secular geneticists like Hermann Muller in the field of bioethics. Substantive, contentful, theologically informed accounts of religion (and even spirituality) were quickly replaced with instrumentalist accounts focusing on the potential positive effects of religion or spirituality on health outcomes or the use of spirituality to instrumentally manage patient care. This becomes clearest when spirituality itself is deemed "unhealthy." As with Pargament earlier, Christina Puchalski also maintains that one can differentiate between "'positive' versus 'negative' spirituality":

> [If] spiritual issues don't really seem to be important, then I may not do anything with that content. But if someone comes in and says something that I hear as a warning sign, I might want to refer to a trained chaplain to help sort that out. For example, a person may see God as punitive and spiritual assessment may allow me to make a link between this attitude and the patient's not wanting to take medicines, or not taking care of him or herself.[62]

Spirituality becomes an occasion for intervention—in other words, its content becomes important—when it subverts the goals of medicine.[63]

The endpoint of this logic of instrumentality is a consumerist or commodified approach to spirituality and religious practice. Health care itself is located in an ever increasingly consumerist culture. Not surprisingly, the increase in interest in spirituality over the past decade or so has paralleled the trend toward commodification of medicine itself. As Joel Shuman and Keith Meador have incisively noted:

> The movement in contemporary North American culture for a more religious medicine has more to do with the fact that both religion and medicine have become phenomena shaped by the consumerist ethos of late modernity. . . . Religion and medicine are, in contemporary North American culture, means of achieving desirable goods external to their practice; both are increasingly viewed as means for self-interested individuals to attain the nearly universally desirable commodity that is individual health. Health is thus . . . to borrow the language of Marxist critique, fetishized, meaning it is valued, pursued, and exchanged without reference to the persons or communities who produce it or to its proper place in a hierarchy of goods of a society committed of pursuing a substantive account of human flourishing.[64]

We find in the literature under consideration here a similar fetishization of spirituality and religious practices. Unmoored from their traditional or communal sources, spiritual or religious practices became services and coping options among which patients might choose—pastoral counseling, meditation, energy work, chapel service, Reiki, Therapeutic Touch, yoga, anointing. Even anointing has not been immune; to some it has seemed offensive to limit anointing to Christians, when it ought rather be available to anyone who wants to experience the comforting touch of oil in the company of significant others to make the "feel bad" places in their bodies "feel good."[65] Patients may choose some, all, or most importantly, *none* of the above.[66]

George Engel was, of course, a psychiatrist. Bishop notes that, in the 1970s, psychiatry (like medicine) was in crisis. Psychiatrists, apparently, were not sure "whether the 'categories of human distress' that they treat are properly considered 'disease,'"[67] lacking as they did at the time an identifiable biological basis. Somewhat surprisingly, Engel targets Christianity as the course of the problems with reductionistic, technological medicine. As Bishop notes:

> Engel does not repudiate Western science; he merely opposes the reductive nature of Western medicine. Rather than arguing that science itself is reductive, Engel lays the blame at the feet of a medical science that has been infected by a Christian dualism. The purported mind/body dualism of Christianity defines the body as a mechanism separate from the mind or soul, resulting, he argues, in a science that places too much emphasis on the physical body and too little on the psyche or on society.[68]

The invention of the biopsychosocialspiritual model was therefore not just a proposed solution to a crisis in medicine and psychiatry, nor was it solely a masked move to totalize the jurisdiction of medicine: via the subterfuge of encompassing spirituality, the biopsychosocialspiritual model became a decisive weapon in the ongoing conflict between religion and the Masters of Suspicion who founded the field of psychiatry. Consequently, it is not accidental that most of the research and writing in the field of spirituality and medicine is conducted by persons located within the disciplines of psychiatry, psychology, and counseling, and that spirituality and religion are, ultimately, reduced to psychological modes of coping. As medical ethics saved the life of philosophy, it could be argued that spirituality—as a component of the biopsychosocialspiritual model of medicine—played a key role in ousting religion and saving the life of psychiatry, catalyzing its promotion to a mode of biopower, finally coequal with its medical counterparts.[69]

BEYOND BIOPOLITICS: THE EMBODIED POLITICS OF RELIGIOUS PRACTICES

It is plausible, thus, to suggest that the field of spirituality and medicine has become part of the biopolitical matrix of medicine. As long as spirituality facilitates medicine's efficiency in serving the ends of the social order, it will be welcomed within the halls of the modern medical center. As long as it reproduces radically individualized consumers, who understand themselves as primarily autonomous choosers or decision makers, and stays in its private, interiorized, subjective space, it will be considered legitimate and perhaps a necessary partner. If it does not, flags immediately go up.

We find such flags in an essay by Stephen Post, Christina Puchalski, and David Larson entitled "Physicians and Patient Spirituality: Professional Boundaries, Competency, and Ethics." As the title suggests, they here grapple with the thorny issues of "professional boundaries"—a key question in the always-conflicted process of biopolitical disciplinary formation.[70] The issue with which they grapple is a "serious ethical question [pertaining to] the actions of physicians who also wish to act as pastoral caregivers."[71] In a deeply revelatory passage, they suggest:

> [I]t is a general mandate of modern developed societies to keep professional roles separate. For example, one does not expect the clergy person who is also a licensed physician to wear his or her pastoral garb in the clinic when functioning as a clinician, nor the white physician's coat at religious service. (Yet the physician-minister or the physician who intends to proselytize, when serving in developing countries or in health care settings that are religious and clearly advertise themselves as such, may merge roles without controversy.) . . .
>
> The pressure to blur the boundaries between the professions often comes from patients. For example, about half of patients indicate a desire to have physicians pray with them. If this finding is accurate, physicians might need to explain to patients why such activities usually better fall under the pur-

view of competent pastoral care. . . . Over the past three decades, biomedical ethics has focused on demystifying the authority of the paternalistic, "priestly" physician of old, thereby allowing greater patient empowerment through autonomy and self-determination.

Adding a sacred or religious mystique to the power of the physician is suspect. For example, we would not condone a Jesuit medical geneticist who maintains that it is appropriate and "nondirective" to wear his clerical collar when doing reproductive genetic counseling in a non-Roman Catholic health care setting. Nor would we want the clinician in a nonreligious health care setting to raise the question, "Have you accepted the Lord?" Many patients would be confused and rightly offended.[72]

Many would be "*rightly offended*." When it comes to religious practices such as prayer—though not "spirituality"—Post and his colleagues are clearly unsettled by the prospect of fluid boundaries. Health care professionals are enjoined to be particularly vigilant in policing them. Not only might such boundary crossing be confusing; it would be *offensive*. Deeply seated—deeply embodied—sensibilities are at stake here.

Yet not for all. It could be uncontroversial, the authors admit, for a clergy-physician to merge roles in a developing country. "About half of patients" would like their physicians to pray with them. Patients, in other words, are insufficiently "normalized." Thus, it falls to the physician (at least in the United States) to order them rightly, "to explain to [them] why such activities usually better fall under the purview of competent pastoral care."

The passage from Post and colleagues reveals that more is going on in religious practices like anointing the sick than simply "meaning-making" or "coping." Rather, I would suggest that religious practices are equally disciplinary, equally embodied, equally political, but seeking to reproduce not citizens for contemporary society but rather adherents of a different social order, namely, faithful disciples for the church or members of the kingdom of God. Thus, Post and colleagues are quite right to be worried about the permeability of the boundaries where medicine and religious practice meet. A priest in the ICU ought rightly be seen as a bizarre irruption of the church—of an alternative politics—in the domain of medicine. Indeed, practices like anointing are, essentially, practices of resistance. In their concrete, embodied, communal, public materiality, they cannot but resist the philosophical dualisms that shape the space in which they are permitted to operate. Rooted in traditions and understood as ends in themselves, they resist instrumentalization and commodification. And, as oriented toward a radically different *telos*, they potentially provide a concretely embodied means to resist cultural hegemony.

Thus, it is not only the case that the field of spirituality and medicine construes both spirituality and religion in ways deeply counter to normative Christian understandings of itself, of sickness, health, healing, spirituality, religion, divorced from theological contexts of belief, practice, and community—to the point that theologians and religious practices like anointing of the sick can find little if any place in this literature. It is not only the case that the field has failed to consult with those with real theological expertise. It is not only the case that theologians have dropped the ball in seeking to participate in this field.

Rather, they were edged out, just as the theologians were edged out of bioethics. It happened to them unawares, under the most benign and deceptive of auspices—that of making space for patients' religious preferences in the clinical setting as a way of attending to their care, promoting their wholistic healing, and providing meaning in their dying. The agenda, then, is before us. Seeking to infuse the field of spirituality and medicine with more accurate and substantive theological content, with more intellectual rigor regarding the realities of spirituality and religion will not be enough. At stake is a contest of polities, of regimes of truth, waged via the bodies of patients and the populace. Those committed to questions of religion and medicine are challenged to begin to attend in a more careful historical, sociological, and theoretical way to the particular continent historical forces that gave rise to the field of spirituality and medicine, including the political commitments of the particular context in which it arose both within society as well as within the realm of medicine. We are challenged to unmask the arbitrary nature of the field's normative structure as well as the dubious scientific status of many of its claims. Equally, we are challenged to come to a deeper appreciation of political dimensions of religious traditions particularly as they are enacted through embodied engagement with adherents. It may well be our own failure to understand the power and complexity of our own traditions that enabled their deformed marginalization.

We find this power and complexity, I think, in the very practices of our traditions. In many ways, they speak more powerfully than any analyses, though they speak quietly and we tend not to listen. Such witness is given by John Carmody, whose experience of anointing opened these reflections. For I think in his conclusion he captures precisely this truth, that an embodied practice like anointing the sick is not simply a health technology in service of "meaning," but rather is an embodied politics—a practice by which the sick are claimed or reclaimed by the church. He concludes:

> Lying in my narrow hospital bed, feeling the oil of gladness and healing, I knew I had little time. More importantly, though, I felt, by a wondrous grace, that this was the first time in my effective memory that the church . . . was praying for me individually, by name, to deal with painful circumstances, suffering, and needs uniquely my own. . . .
>
> [With anointing,] [s]omething maternal really did appear. I truly felt taken to the bosom of a holy family that cared for me. It knew about my muscle spasms and my dismal prognosis. It loved me despite my many manifest failings and my worst secret sins. . . . [I]t was a community of prayer, offering the praise and petition that have always been its primary reason to be. And, for what seemed to me to be the first time, I, little John, weak John, competent John, mixed-up John, strong John, very sick John had a name in this community. My pain grieved it. My dying would sadden and diminish it. I mattered. . . . [T]he church at prayer in my anointing said, . . . "Come close, into our embrace. Become part of the communion of saints as we intercede for you to God."[73]

In anointing, John Carmody found himself reconciled to his mother, the church.

The practice of anointing, then, ought well be seen as deeply subversive of the contemporary configuration of spirituality and medicine, and maybe even of medicine itself. The sacrament of anointing is, indeed, a practice through which patients, families, and sometimes even health professionals find comfort, meaning, and strength to cope with their situation. But more importantly, in the sacrament of anointing of the sick, the church walks into the clinic and claims its own. As the church, as an institutional political body, it cannot help but to challenge the biopolitics of medicine—to break through the well-policed boundaries that not only keep spirituality in the service of medicine but that discipline patients in service of ends not their own. As such, anointing might prove not only to be subversive of spirituality and medicine; it might indeed be its salvation.

NOTES

1. This chapter is a revised and expanded version of papers entitled "*Anointing* the Sick?: Practicing Religion in the Clinical Context," presented at the annual meeting of the American Society of Bioethics and Humanities, October 2004, and at the Duke University Center for Spirituality and Health, May 6, 2010.
2. John Carmody, "Meeting My Mother Again," *Commonweal* 121, no. 5 (1994): 30.
3. For a more nuanced account of these histories that challenge conventional wisdom about the conflict between science/medicine and religion, see Gunter Risse, *Mending Bodies, Saving Souls: A History of Hospitals* (New York: Oxford University Press, 1999); Gary B. Ferngren, *Medicine and Health Care in Early Christianity* (Baltimore: Johns Hopkins University Press, 2009); Christopher J. Kaufman, *Ministry and Meaning: A Religious History of Catholic Healthcare in the United States* (New York: Crossroad Publishing Company, 1995); and Amos Funkenstein, *Theology and the Scientific Imagination From the Middle Ages to the Seventeenth Century* (Princeton, NJ: Princeton University Press, 1989). It is important to note that the relationship between medicine and religion remains quite vibrant and far less conflictual beyond the borders of the United States as well as within poor communities within our own society.
4. In this chapter, for simplicity and consistency, I will use the phrase "spirituality and medicine" to refer to the broader field that includes attention to spirituality, medicine, health, and sometimes religion.
5. Even within the Christian tradition, the status of the anointing of the sick is a bit ambiguous. It certainly is an ancient practice, witnessed in the New Testament and practiced continuously throughout Christian history. Traditions with formal practices associated with illness and healing admit of a wide range of diversity. At the one end

of the spectrum one finds the Orthodox and Roman Catholics, with highly sacramentalized rituals practiced in various settings (sanctuary, home, hospital). Alternatively, traditions of the more Pentecostal variety have developed practices of "faith healing," less high-church perhaps but no less ritualized. Faith healing traditions at times set themselves against modern medicine, offering prayer as an alternative modality in the medical armamentarium whose efficacy is rendered moot should a sick person avail themselves of contemporary medicine.

6. Andrew Lustig, "Prescribing Prayer?: Say the Rosary & Call Me in the Morning," *Commonweal* 131, no. 8 (April 23, 2004): 7.

7. Elsewhere I have argued that if one studies the Christian tradition carefully, one actually finds an inverse relationship between liturgical involvement, spiritual accomplishment, and health. Sanctity, in fact, can be hazardous to one's health. See "Suffering in Communion with Christ: Sacraments, Dying Faithfully, and End-of-Life Care," in *Living Well and Dying Faithfully: Christian Practices for End-of-Life Care*, ed. John Swinton and Richard Payne (Grand Rapids, MI: Wm. B. Eerdmans Publishers, 2009), 59–85. I would now add to the argument there a reference to one of the fundamental practices of the Christian faith: the preferential option for the poor. As many witness, to live in solidarity with the poor may well mean to find oneself the victim of the structured risks that for the poor are everyday realities—death or morbidity from violence or "accidents," from easily treatable communicable diseases, from malnutrition, parasites, and more.

8. This section will primarily draw from the growing literature on "spirituality and medicine." It will focus on those who advocate for spirituality as a means of enhancing the patient-physician relationship (Christina Puchalski and Anna L. Romer, "Taking a Spiritual History Allows Clinicians to Understand Patients More Fully," *Journal of Palliative Medicine* 3 [2000]: 129–37) or honoring patient autonomy (Stephen G. Post, Christina M. Puchalski, and David B. Larson, "Physicians and Patient Spirituality: Professional Boundaries, Competency, and Ethics," *Annals of Internal Medicine* 132 [2000]: 578–83). As mentioned above, an allied literature advocates attending to spirituality within the domain of medicine because of its effects on health outcomes. For an account of the "religion and health" literature parallel to that offered here, see the lucid and compelling analysis in Joel James Shuman and Keith G. Meador, *Heal Thyself: Spirituality, Medicine, and the Distortion of Christianity* (New York: Oxford University Press, 2003). The parallelism between these two conversations is not accidental, as the latter derives from the former.

9. See Jeffrey P. Bishop, *The Anticipatory Corpse: Medicine, Power, and the Care of the Dying* (Notre Dame, IN: University of Notre Dame Press, 2011), 229.

10. Other binaries could also be discussed, e.g., universal vs. particular. It is worth noting an inversion of these binaries relative to their usual positions of normativity. Within much of the Western tradition, formal and mental/rational constructs were allied with objective, public constructs, and often equally correlated with gender (see Jean Bethke Elshtain's classic work, *Public Man, Private Woman: Women in Social and Political Thought* [Princeton, NJ: Princeton University Press, 1981]). Within the spirituality and medicine literature, however, the formal and mental are paired with subjec-

tive and private. Moreover, without saying as such, this normative pole of the binary wherein lies spirituality also seems overwhelmingly feminine, over against the more "masculine" poles of either religion (concrete, particular, embodied, objective, public) which is disvalued or of medicine (also concrete, particular, embodied, objective, public, true) which is valued. This aspect of the discourse on spirituality and medicine warrants further reflection.

11. Puchalski and Romer, "Taking a Spiritual History," 129. They continue further on: "I have a patient who feels that nature is very important, and she said something like, 'I'm a naturalist, and looking at trees makes me feel really centered and with purpose.' In fact, one of the things she said was that if she were dying, she would want me to refer her to a hospice with a window next to some trees, because that's what gives her meaning and purpose in life. Now, I don't think I would have gotten this information out of a strict psychosocial type of interview" (131). Further examples include: "Spirituality . . . pertains to ultimate meaning and purpose in life" (Post et al., "Physicians and Patient Spirituality," 578); "Religiosity is an expression of faith through the practices of a particular religion or denomination, while the predominant understanding of spirituality is meaning-making" (Thomas St. James O'Connor, Elizabeth Meakes, Pam McCarroll-Butler, Shannon Gadowsky, and Kathleen O'Neill, "Making the Most and Making Sense: Ethnographic Research on Spirituality in Palliative Care," *Journal of Pastoral Care* 51 [1997]: 25–36, quotation on 27); or "The understanding of spirituality has also *evolved*. For example, hospice's original religious definition of spirituality as a relationship with God or a Divine Other has been replaced by a definition of spirituality as the personal and psychological search for meaning" (Timothy P. Daaleman and Larry VandeCreek, "Placing Religion and Spirituality in End-of-Life Care," *JAMA* 284 [2000]: 2514–17, quotation on 2516; emphasis added).

    With regard to the religion and health literature, Shuman and Meador note: "Religiosity is . . . an a priori capacity possessed by every human individual" (*Heal Thyself*, 33). They cite Herbert Benson in this regard: "Apparently, just *having* a strong belief is enough to cause things to happen in our physiology, but this is a very ticklish point. It does seem that just the state of belief, which can emanate from a variety of personal, philosophical, or religious orientations, is itself a powerful force. Does it matter what you believe in? Belief in *something* is crucial. The very force and effectiveness of your personal belief stems from your basic assumptions that your belief matters. If you want to experience the physiological benefits of the Faith Factor and you find you have nothing to believe in, it may be helpful to believe generally in the power of life or perhaps even just in the power of belief itself" (*Beyond the Relaxation Response* [Berkeley, CA: Berkeley University Press, 1985], 81–82).

12. O'Connor et al., "Making the Most and Making Sense," 29; emphasis added.

13. Tomasz R. Okon, "Palliative Care Review: Spiritual, Religious, and Existential Aspects of Palliative Care," *Journal of Palliative Medicine* 8 (2005): 392–414, quotation on 392.

14. Yet see also Shuman and Meador: "So the modern account of religion proffered by the advocates of the new rapprochement turns out not to be theologically neutral at

all, for religion is never religion as such but always a particular religion. The freely chosen, utilitarian religion of individual experience is the particular religion of capitalist high modernity" (*Heal Thyself,* 40).

15. Wilfred McSherry and Keith Cash, "The Language of Spirituality: An Emerging Taxonomy," *International Journal of Nursing Studies* 41 (2004): 151–61, quotations on 152.

16. Christina Puchalski, "Spirituality and Health: The Art of Compassionate Medicine," *Hospital Physician* 37, no. 3 (March 2001): 30–36, quotation on 32.

17. Okon, "Palliative Care Review," 392; emphasis added.

18. Shuman and Meador similarly observe: "Even among those whose work has been concerned mostly with 'traditional religious faith and practice,' the decided emphasis in most of the popular literature on religion and health is on the act of believing and the effects of that act, rather than the particular object of belief. Believing is understood primarily as an act of the human will" (*Heal Thyself,* 33).

19. O'Connor et al., "Making the Most and Making Sense," 27.

20. Sometimes data confound the claims within this literature. As Tomasz Okon notes: "In a recent study respondents were asked to define themselves on a religiosity-spirituality spectrum. Ten percent of respondents described themselves as spiritual and not religious. The majority considered themselves both religious and spiritual, while a quarter described themselves as neither religious nor spiritual" (Okon, "Palliative Care Review," 393, citing Leila Shahabi, Lynda H. Powell, Marc A. Musick, Kenneth I. Pargament, Carl E. Thoresen, David Williams, Lynn Underwood, and Marcia A. Ory, "Correlates of Self-Perceptions of Spirituality in American Adults," *Annals of Behavioral Medicine* 24 [2002]: 59–68). What to make of that latter 25 percent?

21. A similar problem is found in the religion and health literature. Here the objective, external, embodied aspects of religion are largely eliminated and religion is reduced to a mental construct. Per Shuman and Meador: "[T]he central issue is the act of believing. Negative beliefs tend to produce negative outcomes, whereas positive beliefs, regardless of the precise material content of their particular object, tend to produce positive outcomes" (*Heal Thyself,* 34).

22. Gary Shogren, "Will God Heal Us?: A Re-Examination of James 5:14–16a," *Evangelical Quarterly* 61 (1989): 99–108, quotation on 99.

23. For these and similar questions from spiritual assessment instruments, see Okon, "Palliative Care Review," 398, Table 3: Constructs of Religion and Spirituality, Instruments, and Illustrative Phrases.

24. As Shuman and Meador note: Spirituality "has its origins in individual human subjectivity, [therefore] it is fundamentally private and personal. . . . In this sense it is decidedly mystical" (*Heal Thyself,* 35).

25. A stock case in bioethics is the case created by an irrational religious belief: Jehovah's Witnesses and blood transfusions; parents who rely on faith healing; the Roman Catholic position on contraception, sterilization, or abortion; family members' hopes for "miracles"; "religious" objections to organ donation; and so forth. Such cases are never characterized as conflicts over "spirituality."

26. Daniel E. Hall, Harold G. Koenig, and Keith G. Meador, "Conceptualizing 'Religion': How Language Shapes and Constrains Knowledge in the Study of Religion and Health," *Perspectives in Biology and Medicine* 47 (2004): 386–401, quotation on 388.

27. As we will see, spirituality and religion are, in this field, largely reduced to matters of feeling and coping. This is due not only to the Kantian commitments of this field (for whom religion was reduced to morality) but equally to the fact that the field of spirituality and medicine was largely birthed and colonized by those in the psychological disciplines. More on this latter point below.

28. O'Connor et al., "Making the Most and Making Sense," 27, 28.

29. Ibid., 32.

30. "Religion, n." in *OED: Oxford English Dictionary* (online version, December 2011), accessed at http://www.oed.com/view/Entry/161944?redirectedFrom=religion.

31. Ibid.

32. Anne Bradshaw has observed, in the context of transformations in the practice of hospice that occurred in the 1980s and 1990s (the same time frame that saw the development of spirituality and medicine), that "the preponderance of medical and psychosocial techniques seem to support the warning . . . that hospice care may become predominantly a technique for the professional expert to exercise power" ("The Spiritual Dimension of Hospice: The Secularization of an Ideal," *Social Science and Medicine* 43 [1996]: 409–19, quotation on 415).

33. See M. Therese Lysaught, "And Power Corrupts . . . Religion and the Disciplinary Matrix of Bioethics," in *The Handbook of Religion and Bioethics*, ed. David E. Guinn (New York: Oxford University Press, 2006), 93–128; and M. Therese Lysaught, "Docile Bodies: Transnational Research Ethics as Biopolitics," *Journal of Medicine and Philosophy* 34 (2009): 384–408. See also Jeffrey P. Bishop and Fabrice Jotterand, "Bioethics as Biopolitics," *Journal of Medicine and Philosophy* 31 (2006): 205–12.

34. Herbert L. Dreyfus, *Michel Foucault: Beyond Structuralism and Hermeneutics* (Chicago: University of Chicago Press, 1982), xxvi; and Joanne L. Finkelstein, "Biomedicine and Technocratic Power," *The Hastings Center Report* 20, no. 4 (1990): 13–16, quotation on 15.

35. Key works by Foucault here include *Discipline and Punish: The Birth of the Prison*, trans. Alan Sheridan (New York: Pantheon Books, 1977); *The Birth of the Clinic: An Archeology of Medical Perception*, trans. A. M. Sheridan Smith (New York: Pantheon, 1973); *The Order of Things: An Archeology of the Human Sciences* [1970] (New York: Vintage, 1990); and *The Birth of Biopolitics: Lectures at the Collège de France, 1978–1979* (New York: Picador Press, 2010).

36. Foucault refers to this dynamic as "governmentality." Governmentality does not ascribe agency to a class or any specific individuals, although some individuals and groups clearly benefit from a given system of institutionalized discursive practices. These practices are not, *per se*, intentional, nor directly under control of particular individuals or groups. Rather, their power lies in that they are, in Dorothy Smith's words, "pervasive and pervasively interconnected" connecting "extralocal" ruling rela-

tions to local contexts (*Reading the Social: Critique, Theory, and Investigations* [Toronto: University of Toronto Press, 1999], 49).

37. The focal point of Foucault's analyses—be it of the clinic, the asylum, or the prison—is the material reality of *bodies*. Foucault is particularly interested in mapping the ways in which bodies within a particular social space are organized and "produced"—shaped, that is, to perceive and behave in particular ways. Within a biopolitical regime, power will not most often be wielded in an overt, coercive manner. Ideally, individuals come to wield it over themselves. Within a regime of disciplinary power, each person—by internalizing the norms and surveillance of the social order—effectively disciplines herself or himself. As such, this exercise of power can direct individuals to engage in actions that are not necessarily to their advantage. In short, the basic goal of disciplinary power is to take wild, unruly persons and produce persons who are "docile"—persons, in other words, who do not have to be externally policed.

38. George L. Engel, "The Need for a New Medical Model: A Challenge for Biomedicine," *Science* 196 (1977): 129–36.

39. Ironically, Shuman and Meador note: "Modern thought, political and scientific, is notoriously reductive" (10), and "radical individualism" (*Heal Thyself*, 10) is but the outworking of that reductiveness in the realm of anthropology. Might one argue that Engel's heirs and the champions of the radically individualistically private biopsychosocialspiritual model corrected the biological reductionism of medicine with an anthropological reductionism—thereby not solving the problem of reductionism at all?

40. As Arthur W. Frank notes: "Theory needs to apprehend the body as both medium and outcome of social 'body techniques,' and society as both medium and outcome of the sum of these techniques. Body techniques are socially given—individuals may improvise on them but rarely make up any for themselves—but these techniques are only instantiated in their practical use by bodies, *on* bodies. Moreover, these techniques are as much resources *for* bodies as they are constraints *on* them; constraints enable as much as they restrict. . . . People construct and use their bodies, though they do not use them in conditions of their own choosing, and their constructions are overlaid with ideologies" ("For a Sociology of the Body: An Analytical Review," in *The Body: Social Process and Cultural Theory*, ed. Mike Featherstone, Mike Hepworth, and Bryan S. Turner [Newbury Park, CA: Sage Publications, 1991], 36–102, quotation on 47, 48).

41. Bodies, of course, can equally resist, recreate, and transform discourses.

42. An additional dividing practice is the distinction between physical pain and nonphysical (existential/spiritual) pain asserted within this field, with both sorts of pain now being subject to medicalization, either through the form of pharmaceutical or personnel intervention. I thank Tomasz Okon for this observation.

43. Bishop, *Anticipatory Corpse.*

44. Ibid., 238.

45. See Carrie M. Dameron, "Spiritual Assessment Made Easy . . . With Acronyms!," *Journal of Christian Nursing* 22, no. 1 (2005): 14–16. This article is a classic example of this literature in many ways. Dameron begins by noting: "Meeting the patient's spiritual needs is part of daily nursing care, yet many nurses feel uncomfortable performing a spiritual assessment. This is especially difficult when the patient presents no clues to their spiritual/religious preference or has a spiritual belief unfamiliar to the nurse. However, there are simple, easy-to-use assessment tools that can help us quickly assess and plan for spiritual needs. . . . None of the questions impart a religion or belief system onto the patient. These are open-ended questions that ask the patients about their personal spiritual beliefs. It is important for Christians and adherents of other religions to phrase questions in a spiritual assessment in a way that is open and non-judgmental" (14).

46. See Bishop, *Anticipatory Corpse*, 241.

47. Kenneth I. Pargament, Harold G. Koenig, and Lisa M. Perez, "The Many Methods of Religious Coping: Development and Initial Validation of the RCOPE," *Journal of Clinical Psychology* 56 (2000): 519–43. As with a significant number of psychosocial and spiritual assessment instruments, the RCOPE was initially validated in part with college students, a group of predominantly white, single, freshman women. The college student cohort is generally known to lack significant knowledge of their own religious traditions and, at the same time, to often be distancing themselves from the religious traditions of their parents. One might speculate that these general characteristics of college students would be more pronounced at public or largely secular institutions (e.g., Bowling Green State University, Duke University) than they would be at religiously affiliated universities. Intriguingly, Pergament and associates find that the RCOPE "proved to be applicable to populations with different levels of religiousness, with different problems, and at different ends of the adult life span" (538)—namely, equally applicable to college students and hospitalized elderly persons, many with quite severe, likely terminal illnesses. Given the necessarily different relationships with their religious traditions necessitated by (roughly) fifty years of lived religion and life events, this finding is quite astounding. This finding likely speaks more to the assumptions built into the instrument than to the differential realities of lived religiosity.

48. Dameron, *Spiritual Assessment Made Easy*, 15.

49. Ibid., 14.

50. Pargament et al., "The Many Methods of Religious Coping," 524.

51. Kyle B. Brothers, "Coping with Religious Coping," *Virtual Mentor* 11 (2009): 767–71, quotation 768.

52. "As one might expect in a culture where religiosity is at once ubiquitous, malleable, and radically individualized, the deity—or more frequently 'faith' or simply 'spirituality'—is often invoked as a means to achieve a variety of ends that are determined by forces of the broader culture" (Shuman and Meador, *Heal Thyself*, 9).

53. As Joanne Finkelstein notes: "It is principally through discourse, that is, through the ways in which systems of knowledge are established, expectations of human abilities

discussed, and subjects and practices described in the working literature of a professional group, that the 'normal' is defined" ("Biomedicine and Technocratic Power," 15).

54. Bishop, *Anticipatory Corpse*, 228.

55. My account of bioethics as biopolitics in "And Power Corrupts . . ." did not attend sufficiently to the role of political economy in biopolitics, a point elucidated for me in Foucault's *The Birth of Biopolitics*. Any account of the biopolitical nature of bioethics, and of spirituality and medicine, must necessarily attend to the political economy of the field as well.

56. See Daniel Callahan, "Religion and the Secularization of Bioethics," *The Hastings Center Report* 20 (1990): S2–4, and the rest of the special supplement on religion and bioethics in that same issue; Janine Marie Idziak, "Theology and the Discipline of Bioethics," *Bioethics Forum* 8, no. 3 (1992): 13–17; and Allen Verhey, *Religion and Medical Ethics: Looking Back, Looking Forward* (Grand Rapids, MI: Wm. B. Eerdmans Publishers, 1996), particularly the essay by Stephen E. Lammers, "The Marginalization of Religious Voices in Bioethics," 19–43.

57. Kevin W. Wildes, "Religion in Bioethics: A Rebirth," *Christian Bioethics* 8 (2002): 163–74, quotation on 163, 168.

58. A longer argument would, of course, plot the contingent historical forces and political commitments that created the radical separation between the religious and the public/political, which created religious belief as a radically private, subjective, individual thing. William T. Cavanaugh's work on the sixteenth-century wars of religion (first outlined in his essay "'A Fire Strong Enough to Consume the House': The Wars of Religion and the Rise of the State," *Modern Theology* 11 [1995]: 397–420; and then developed more fully in his recent book *Theopolitical Imagination: Christian Practices of Space and Time* [London: T&T Clark, 2002]) provides this account. Here he demonstrates how the wars of "religion" were not so much about "religion"—they were about the reconfiguration and consolidation of new forms of political power—but that this political process was masked by the use of rhetoric about "religion" which cast "religion" as this terribly divisive and violence-inciting thing that must therefore, for peace and the public good, be relegated to the realm of the private. Once religion is banished to the private realm—interiorized, disembodied, disincorporated—Freud (the negative reading of religion) or James (the experiential expressivist) follows, giving rise on the one hand to a contentless "universal spirituality" in the public realm or to "psychologism" in the realm of medicine.

59. Unlike spirituality, certain human persons can be deemed to lack autonomy, but autonomous persons, per the above account, cannot be without spirituality within this construct, even if they autonomously deny or reject it!

60. John H. Evans, *Playing God?: Human Genetic Engineering and the Rationalization of Public Bioethical Debate* (Chicago: University of Chicago Press, 2002).

61. Quoted from the prologue to the present book (Jeff Levin, "The Intersection of Spirituality, Theology, and Health," in *Healing to All Their Flesh: Jewish and Christian Perspectives on Spirituality, Theology, and Health*, ed. Jeff Levin and Keith G. Meador (West Conshohocken, PA: Templeton Press, 2012), 000.

62. Quotation from Anna L. Romer, "Taking a Spiritual History Allows Clinicians to Understand Patients More Fully: An Interview with Dr. Christina Puchalski," *Innovations in End-of-Life Care* 1, no. 6 (1999); accessed at http://www2.edc.org/lastacts/archives/archivesNov99/featureinn.asp.

63. Cf. Daaleman and VandeCreek, "Placing Religion and Spirituality in End-of-Life Care": "Religion-based ethics can both facilitate and impede clinical decision-making" (2514). It seems, however, that if creating a space for spirituality in the clinical setting is about fostering patient autonomy, judgments about "positive" and "negative" spirituality would be unwarranted. This slip on Puchalski's part betrays the deeper biopolitical motive of spirituality and medicine. Shuman and Meador aptly identify this as a utilitarian approach to spirituality: if it is useful, it should be pursued; if it would lead to negative health or well-being outcomes, it should be avoided (*Heal Thyself*, 37). As in bioethics, utilitarianism is hard to overcome, even with regard to spirituality.

64. Shuman and Meador, *Heal Thyself*, 6.

65. Jerome W. Berryman, "The Rite of Anointing and the Pastoral Care of Sick Children," in *The Sacred Play of Children*, ed. Diane Apostolos-Cappadona (New York: Seabury Press, 1983): 63–77.

66. The chaplain members of the interdisciplinary care team are the only members that generally are optional; those patients who are not interested in addressing the spiritual dimensions of their illness or dying process are not required to do so. Foregoing interaction with the physician, nurse, or social worker is far more difficult.

67. Bishop, *Anticipatory Corpse*, 229.

68. Ibid., 234.

69. See Stephen Toulmin's now classic article, "How Medicine Saved the Life of Ethics," in *New Directions in Ethics: The Challenge of Applied Ethics*, ed. Joseph P. DeMarco and Richard M. Fox (New York: Routledge and Kegan Paul, 1986), 265–81. By "ethics," here, Toulmin is referring to secular analytic philosophy.

70. The disjunct between spirituality and religiosity is reinforced professionally. O'Connor and associates note: "Religious needs are best handled by a competent person from the patient's religious faith group. . . . Spiritual needs [on the other hand] can be handled by competent health-care professionals from a variety of disciplines" ("Making the Most and Making Sense," 28). Puchalski's work, of course, is designed precisely to encourage health care professionals to develop this competency.

71. Post et al., "Physicians and Patient Spirituality," 581.

72. Ibid.

73. Carmody, "Meeting My Mother Again," 30.

STEPHEN G. POST

8. THE ONTOLOGICAL GENERALITY IN SPIRITUALITY AND HEALTH

Among the most embarrassing statements a researcher can make is that unqualified "religion is good for health." Religion can be very healthy or very unhealthy, and this must be sorted out with more nuance. Moreover, when religion is healthy, what religion are we speaking of, under what conditions, and what is it about that religion that is salutogenic? Moreover, is health an ultimate or penultimate value in the particular tradition itself? Jeff Levin has wisdom to offer. In his article entitled "'And Let Us Make a Name': Reflections on the Future of the Religion and Health Field," published in *Journal of Religion and Health* in 2009, he writes, "Religion, generally speaking, may fill a deep void in people's lives or be harmful to many people's minds and souls, and it may be a positive force in human history or a destructive one, but surely epidemiologic research studies tell us little at all one way or the other about such profound matters."[1]

The too-easy assertion of an association between religion and health is quite embarrassing, as the person on the street knows from reading the papers about a Christian fundamentalist in Norway who shot down more than ninety children at a summer camp after blowing up a government building, all in the name of Christ, or about a small group of believers-in-something in San Diego who packed suitcases, castrated themselves, and drank lethal poison in order to ascend to the Hale-Bopp Comet. The quantitative epidemiologist of religion and health who makes easy assertions about an association does not quite sound serious, even if there is some association to be found from pouring over large population databases of regular worshippers, presumably in established churches and synagogues.

The field of health, spirituality, and religion is not entirely healthy. It has become insular and technocratic, perhaps the inevitable result of the absence of creative visionary dialogue between narrowly trained epidemiologists or other researchers and world-class theological and spiritual minds who can ask "big" interpretive questions. It is a field that is conceptually somewhat frozen because without a major "broaden and build" mind-set of dialogue with spiritual and theological minds, there is little or no depth of interpretation.

Tremendous resources have been pumped into the field of religion and health. We learned that often very sick people cope with illness through drawing on faith, just as Kierkegaard observed long ago in his discussions of anxiety, finitude, and lack of control.[2] We know that many people in hospitals want pastoral care and a spiritual history available to them. We assert that people who are regular worshippers live a little longer and have lower depression. There are a few other obvious things we know, vaguely, but we have not learned much that would be unexpected.

When a claim about "religion" contributing to health or longevity is made, we need to acknowledge that this is superficial, partly because religion can be a very destructive force as well. Researchers have usually not acknowledged the ambivalence that most people have about "religion," which can bring out the very best and the very worst in adherents. This lacuna has trivialized the field. Moreover, "religion" is such a weak and entirely vague variable as to be nearly meaningless. We need to focus on particular religions and spiritualities in their differences.

What is it that any association between religion and health is revealing? Is it the social capital in particular spiritualities and religions that is at work? Is it the disinhibition of compassion and altruism in this organized community of generativity that is at work? Is it faith in God (in those religions that believe in such)? Is it related to the positive psychology inherent in a given spirituality or religion as a venue for hope, gratitude, love, awe, faith, joy, courage, etc.? If so, are some spiritualities and religions better positive-psychology venues than others? Is religion *sui generis*, or merely a supermarket with lots of shelves full of needed emotional supports and strengths? Is it that marriages tend to last longer in certain religious communities? Is it the diet and stewardship of the body that is at work? Is it spirituality in the sense of filling a void in the human heart that only "Something More" can fill? Is it self-control that is operative?

I will suggest a theological interpretive framework herein under the rubric of the *Ontological Generality*. This framework will be applied in an effort to provide a theological groundwork with which to interpret any and all purported associations between spirituality and health more meaningfully. I have coined the term "Ontological Generality" to capture a perennial aspect of theological anthropology. The term refers to the *communitas* between self, others, and a Higher Power in which our full flourishing as individuals is possible. However, it must be recognized that many spiritualities and religions fail miserably at creating communities grounded in the Ontological Generality, and they therefore would not be expected to have notable benefits.

THE ONTOLOGICAL GENERALITY

Most spiritualities posit the need for attachment between self and others, and between self and a Higher Power. The full being of the human agent lies not in the isolated monad, nor even in the relational dyad of self and other, but in the triadic structure of God, self, and other. For example, Jesus of Nazareth drew on Jewish tradition in teaching that human flourishing lies in the fulfilling of a double-love commandment:

> "You shall love the Lord your God with all your heart, and with all your soul, and with all your mind." This is the first and great commandment. And the second is like to it: "You shall love your neighbor as yourself." On these two commandments hang all the law and the prophets.[3]

Human abundance and well-being lie in the love of God, neighbor, and self. Well-being does not lie in the love of self alone, or in the love of God alone, or in the love of neighbor alone. The three must be conjoined in a triadic community of being that defines the Ontological Generality. It would be difficult to find a theologian who has not asserted this Ontological Generality in some fashion, for its disruption constitutes incompleteness (or "fallenness" or "sin"), and its restoration constitutes spiritual flourishing. It is abundantly clear from the Gospels that Jesus modeled this restored state of triadic being, and that he maintained this state despite torture and crucifixion, wherein lies one aspect of his redemptive power.

Now this Ontological Generality is the foundation not just of the Abrahamic faiths, but of most all religions, faiths, and spiritualities however differently a Higher Power might be described. The Hindus will state that their gods are not unlike the Trinity, the three-in-one, and the Native Americans will point to the Great Spirit. However articulated within a cultural system, the mystical triadic structure of "I" in relation to "Thou" at the horizontal and vertical levels of self, other, and God seems nearly universal, if not entirely so.

As a Christian thinker, I assert that Jesus of Nazareth lived every moment of his life in profound love of God, of neighbor, and of self, relationally considered. One discerns this in the depth of his heartfelt prayers, in his astonishing forgiving and healing love of those around him, and in his carrying himself with grace and dignity in thought, word, and action.

Theologically, I will then assert that "health," or "flourishing," or "well-being" are ultimately only fully available in the context of genuine *communitas* between God, self, and other. This does not mean that individuals cannot achieve lesser but significant degrees of flourishing outside of this triadic structure, nor does it mean that individuals who are authentically engaged in such *communitas* formed around the Ontological Generality will not be susceptible to severe diagnoses of disease early in life, or to fatal or disabling accidents and the like. However, as a gross generalization, those who abide in the love of the Ontological

Generality will cultivate positive spiritual emotions such as joy, hope, faith, gratitude, and kindness; they will be more shielded from destructive, vengeful, and hostile emotions; they will find more resilience in the face of adversity; they will live lives of higher purpose and calling that will protect them from falling into violent, life-shortening, antisocial activities; and they will have a deeper sense of self-stewardship because their lives are understood as valued by both God and neighbor.

In this chapter, I will discuss health in relation to the Ontological Generality, which includes both its horizontal (self and other) and vertical dimensions (self and God) working synergistically and simultaneously. But I will also assert that "religion" in relation to health is almost, but not quite, a meaningless variable, and that any generalizations about an association between religion and health are in real fact difficult to make because the Ontological Generality is so badly distorted in the filters of so many religious communities. It is really, then, only possible to speak meaningfully of health in relation to a particular spiritual or religious tradition as lived and practiced. After all, every person who reads the papers knows that some religions, faiths, and spiritualities are destructive, suicidal, or masochistic snake pits providing a blank check for personality disorders, replete with every distortion of whatever universal truths they might use to camouflage wanton manipulations and the sheer will to power. This reality means that any statements about human health and religion must be very carefully limited and circumscribed.

These quantitative epidemiologists are not all wrong. Where the Ontological Generality manifests in relatively undistorted fashion there should be some positive association between religion and health, although even here, the distinction between "intrinsic" (heartfelt spirituality) and "extrinsic" (involvement for purposes of social capital) religiosity cannot be lost sight of. Yet another caveat is needed: while health is a value within the context of the Ontological Generality, it is regrettably the case that in a disordered and dismembered world many who adhere profoundly to the Ontological Generality will almost surely experience considerable unrest, including the possibility of significant harm. I wish I could say that everyone who tries to abide in the love of the Ontological Generality receives accolades and praise, but, regrettably, this is far from true. The Ontological Generality does very generally contribute to health at the statistical level, but it also gives rise to its martyrs.

We do see the association between health and the Ontological Generality shine through in some astonishing *particular* religious contexts where health is fragile. Perhaps the most powerful example of this is Alcoholics Anonymous, which I will explore as a prototype that points toward a more generalizable model that will be explored subsequently.

ALCOHOLICS ANONYMOUS AS A PROTOTYPICAL EXAMPLE OF HEALING THROUGH ADHERENCE TO THE ONTOLOGICAL GENERALITY

The Ontological Generality is powerfully exemplified with respect to recovery and health by Alcoholics Anonymous (AA). If the Ontological Generality is in fact true, AA should be viewed as a prototype of healing that provides broad insights into the current inability of secularized cultures to generate much flourishing. The triadic flow of mutual love that constitutes the inner dynamic of the Ontological Generality is restorative not only for the addict, but for all of us. The Ontological Generality always includes both a horizontal (self and other) component and a vertical (self and God) component. We would thus expect to see some health benefits along both relational axes, but greater benefits when these are in synergy.

The Twelve Steps are essentially a "how to" articulation of the Ontological Generality. First, there is an acknowledgment that the agent is powerless to solve this addiction alone, and that only a "Higher Power" can (Steps One, Two, and Three). Second, there is a precise spiritual-moral confession of past wrongs committed, a willingness to have God remove our moral defects, an active effort to make apologies and amends wherever plausible (with elements of forgiveness and reconciliation), and a readiness to engage in such continued moral inventory (Steps Four, Five, Six, Seven, Eight, Nine, and Ten). Third, there is a deepened life of prayer and meditation focused on doing God's will rather than our own (Step Eleven). Fourth, there is an active effort to serve other alcoholics by witnessing to these steps and modeling them in practice. In practice, these elements, while building on one another, do not follow in a rigidly sequential fashion. Different individuals will implement these steps with different emphases and timing. Service to others can start quickly in very practical ways, for it allows a sense of active agency and purpose that can be extremely helpful to the helper. Spirituality may come a little later with growing acculturation to the AA group. Some members of AA will for a while resist much moral inventory as their insights into their behavior develop. Some will be more easily inclined to spirituality or talk of a Higher Power. Thus, while the Twelve Steps are ordered, it would be too limiting to suggest that in practice they must be engaged in sequentially.

The Twelve Steps assert that little good can happen in the life of an alcoholic until a community is established between self, other, and God. The dynamic of a Higher Power has always been considered a crucial aspect of recovery. Columnist David Brooks of the *New York Times* quotes the self-reported experience of Bill W., not previously a believer, as he experienced a white light that he perceived as the presence of God. He described what occurred in his hospital room at a New York City detox center on his fourth day of treatment: "It seemed to me, in the mind's eye, that I was on a mountain and a wind not of air but of spirit was blowing. And then it burst upon me that I was a free man."[4] Bill W. never drank again after that spiritual experience of December 14, 1934. But Bill W. also came to realize that he could never recover without the additional element of helping other alcoholics like himself in the context of mutual aid.

The Ontological Generality is of course antithetical to psychological narcissism (or what moralists call "solipsism" or theologians call "sin"). *Alcoholics Anonymous*, subtitled, *The Story of How Many Thousands of Men and Women Have Recovered from Alcoholism,*[5] is called the *Big Book* in AA circles. First printed in 1939 (now in its 2001 fourth edition), the opening segment of this spiritual-moral treatment manual begins with the words, "We of Alcoholics Anonymous."[6] The essence of the program is captured in the passage, "We work out our solution on the *spiritual as well as an altruistic plane* [emphasis added]...."[7] Nowhere is the word "I" to be found, because self-preoccupation is considered the root of the problem. Grandiosity is replaced by anonymity and humility. Any solution lies in the "we" of fellowship centered on a Higher Power, and the recognition that "I" cannot rescue myself.[8] As the *Big Book* emphasizes, "Selfishness—self-centeredness! That, we think, is the root of our troubles."[9] We must be rid of this by becoming "less and less interested in ourselves, our little plans and designs,"[10] and more interested in what we can "contribute to life."[11] Moreover, "our very lives, as ex-problem drinkers, depend upon our constant thought of others and how we may help their needs."[12] Still, our helping others in need must be based in "*a sincere desire to be helpful* [emphasis added]."[13] All of this prosociality, however, is clearly positioned under the sacred canopy of a Higher Power.

In the most general terms, recovery as captured in the Twelve Steps involves a shift in thought, emotion, and activity away from self and toward others and God. It is a process well described by Martin Buber as a shift from "I-It" to "I-Thou." The alcoholic has suffered from the delusion that he or she is the center of the universe, that the planets revolve around that center, and as a consequence he or she has related to others only insofar as they satisfy his or her own little plans and agendas. But "I-Thou" involves a holistic transformation facilitated and supported in a community. "I" am not the center of the universe, but we are.

As stated, AA understands that the alcoholic must have a connection to a Higher Power, which alone is powerful enough to fill the void that was previously flooded with alcohol. Not everyone in AA is equally spiritual, and only some report the intense spiritual experience like that of Bill W. Yet there is a great deal of spirituality among AA members. Some come into AA with a strong spiritual history that is still vital and active in their daily lives. Others come in no longer spiritual or religious, but having been so earlier in life. There are those who have never been spiritually or religiously engaged in the past, but their involvement with AA brings them to spirituality as they are affirmed and seek to acculturate to this healing community.

This spirituality achieves several important things. First, such a Higher Power functions to create an absolute quality to abstinence, which becomes more than a mere human contrivance or a matter of "relative" value. Abstinence is therefore nonnegotiable. Second, reliance on a Higher Power takes the place of alcohol in filling the emptiness or incompleteness within. This theme of spiritual emptiness and the misplaced efforts to find fulfillment through things other than God's love can be found in the writings of Western spirituality from the fourth century. *Third*, this spirituality frees the self to concentrate on contrition and service.

Moral inventory, offering apologies, and making amends also lie in the center of the Twelve Steps. The alcoholic is often shockingly unconcerned about the damage that he or she inflicts on others. Recovery thus involves a major moral transformation. When an alcoholic shares his dark secrets and past experiences with alcohol, he reaches a fellow sufferer like "no one else can."[14] Transforming past mistakes to good (i.e., redemption) also occurs when an alcoholic faces the wreckage of his past and mends the bridges he burned with others. Progress is made by the daily pruning of egocentrism: "Selfishness—self-centeredness! That, we think, is the root of our troubles."[15] And further, "above everything, we alcoholics must be rid of this selfishness. We must, or it kills us!"[16] The *Big Book* refers to selfish resentment, dishonesty, self-seeking, and unkindness, among other manifestations.

Prayer and meditation are prescribed as spiritual practices necessary to remain "in contact" with a Higher Power and the will of God for our lives.

The Twelfth Step, "having had a spiritual awakening as the result of these steps, we tried to carry this message to alcoholics, and to practice these principles in all our affairs,"[17] is vital. The *Big Book* is abundantly clear: "Our very lives, as ex-problem drinkers, depend upon our constant thought of others and how we may help meet their needs."[18] The word *constant* indicates that this concern with helping other drinkers must become an enduring daily practice to keep the disease in remission. AA literature teaches the alcoholic to apply the spiritual principle of service in all his affairs, to practice "tolerance, patience and good will toward all men,"[19] and to "place the welfare of other people ahead of his own."[20] The preceding eleven steps must be "accompanied by self sacrifice and unselfish, constructive action."[21] Members of AA understand that as they help other alcoholics, they also help themselves. This principle is clear in the purpose statement of AA: "Our primary purpose is to stay sober and help other alcoholics to achieve sobriety."[22] The relevant aphorism is: "If you help someone up the hill, you get closer yourself." There is a deep sense of purpose in such a role, and a powerful new self-identity as a "wounded healer," one who assists others from one's reservoir of firsthand knowledge.

The Twelve Steps have been practiced daily in the lives of recovering alcoholics since 1935. It is curious that empirical support for the link between helping others and staying sober first manifested only in 2004.[23] Using data from a prospective study called Project MATCH, one of the largest clinical trials in alcohol research, Pagano and colleagues found that alcoholics who helped others during chemical dependency treatment were more likely to be sober in the following twelve months. Specifically, 40 percent of those who helped other alcoholics avoided taking a drink in the twelve months that followed a three-month chemical dependency treatment period, in comparison to 22 percent of those not helping.

Dr. Maria E. Pagano led the study of helping behaviors of alcoholics with a range of sixteen to twenty-five years of continuous abstinence from alcohol. While helping others in general was rated as significant in contribution to sobriety, considerably higher benefits came from increased helping of other alcoholics in the context of Alcoholics Anonymous.[24] Earlier, she and her colleagues examined the relationship between helping other alcoholics to recover (the Twelfth Step) and relapse in the year following treatment.[25] The data, from Project MATCH, examined different treatment options for alcoholics and evaluated their efficacy in preventing relapse. Two measures of helping other alcoholics in Alcoholics Anonymous (being a sponsor and having completed the Twelfth Step) were isolated from the data. Proportional hazards regressions were used to separate these variables from the number of AA meetings attended during the period. The authors found that "those who were helping were significantly less likely to relapse in the year following treatment. . . ."[26] Among those who helped other alcoholics (8 percent of the study population), 40 percent avoided taking a drink in the year following treatment; only 22 percent of those not helping had the same outcome. Imagine, helping others doubles the likelihood of recovery from alcoholism in a one-year period!

Service can take many forms, one of which is sponsoring another member into AA and the Twelve Steps. Sponsoring is typically not done until the sponsor has been sober and a member of AA for a year or more, since sponsoring is a very significant responsibility and form of service. But service can involve all the small things needed to make an AA meeting succeed, from being a greeter at the door to cleaning up the room after a meeting. A key aspect of service is being willing to give one's testimony at an AA meeting in order to inspire others and contribute to the group ethos. It is possible to visit other alcoholics in detox clinics or in prisons, or simply to provide some companionship and attentive listening to a friend or colleague who may be struggling with alcoholism. It does seem clear that the potency of benefits for those engaged in service is greater when they are serving another alcoholic,[27] and this is certainly the emphasis in AA. But still, service "in all our affairs" is stressed in the Twelfth Step, and there are less pronounced benefits in serving others outside of AA in general helpful behaviors.

The Twelve Steps, then, present a format for recovery based on the Ontological Generality that has come to the rescue of a great many alcoholics around the world. But this approach to recovery and health has not made many inroads into other recovery programs run in professional settings. Indeed, professionals still lack a deep understanding of why a grassroots mutual aid program like AA is remarkably effective. Might the Ontological Generality be applicable to many other areas of recovery and prevention, from obesity and depression to heart disease and anxiety? Might it be relevant to all contexts of a real association between spirituality and health?

RELIGION AND HEALTH AS FULLY INTERPRETABLE IN LIGHT OF THE ONTOLOGICAL GENERALITY

We will not here summarize the various epidemiologic studies of the association between religious attendance and health, many of which examine a crude "religion" variable that happens to be included in some large population study. These numerous studies are somewhat useful in pointing out that there is something about being a regular church worshipper that is associated with mainly lower depression rates and some moderate reduction in mortality rates. But what is it within "religion" that is actually really at work? The Ontological Generality would suggest that a number of dynamics are at work in a synergy, including:

The Experience of Divine Love

By this theory, only a reconciliation with God completes human nature and creates an internal homeostasis. We humans have a God-shaped hole that only God can fill. This is the view taken by organizations such as AA, where healing occurs through reliance on a Higher Power, however understood. Augustine spoke of a rest that can only be found in God, and most Western theology has placed *eudaimonia* not in worldly *felicitas* but in the *viseo Dei*. We cannot feel complete or whole, we cannot feel serene or at rest, when we try to find happiness in anything that is created. We find full happiness in knowing and loving God.

The Care of the Self

One triad of the Ontological Generality is the care of the self. We live in a culture and a time when the care of the self is floundering at many levels outside of the love of God and neighbor. It may be difficult to care for self unless there are reasons beyond the self to do so. The care of the self within the Ontological Generality is a stewardship that is grounded in a deep appreciation for the love one receives from God and others, which so greatly enhances one's sense of significance and dignity. Why abide by healthy lifestyle behaviors and refrain from self-harm if one's life is focused merely on self? The self is not meaningful enough to care for itself. Salutogenic meaning in the deep sense that one's life is more than an exercise in fleeting emptiness is found in the mutual love of the Ontological Generality.

Spiritualities and religions can enhance health and prevent disease through the care of the self (e.g., self-control in diet and sexual activity; the eradication of smoking and substance abuse; physical exercise and other positive health practices; nonviolence), but this is care grounded in the Ontological Generality. We know that Seventh-Day Adventists are particularly long-lived, that Judaism includes its dietary and other regulations, etc. To select a purely symbolic number, let us say that 95 percent of the health benefits of spirituality and religion have to do with the care of the self, and when looked at globally, this is probably the most significant worldwide contribution that spirituality and religion make to the human condition.

We need a global program in spiritual flourishing and the health of body, mind, culture, and society. Let us reconceptualize and re-create the field anew at a global preventive level. Can we really begin to understand how certain spiritualities and religions do promote health in certain regions of the globe? Is there a future in which the value of the care of the self and the care of the other under a sacred canopy can be much better appreciated, cultivated, and acknowledged? Prevention and responsibility are the future.

Has there been a deterioration in the care of the self in the United States, or in other countries across the globe? What are the deeper spiritual, cultural, individual, and community underpinnings of good care of the self? What is the history of self-care? Have the traditions of self-care broken down? Are there features of modern society that work against self-care? Is the Ontological Generality our hope for a paradigm shift that can bring down health care costs through prevention and self-care?

The care of the self is a topic that no health care reform program can afford to ignore. It might be estimated that about a third of health care expenditures in the United States result from patient noncompliance (or nonadherence), and another third from destructive and self-destructive behaviors of all kinds. Many people take little or no responsibility for their health, expecting physicians to fix with a pill problems rooted in long-standing unhealthy behaviors. Everyone wants access to health care, but this will never succeed without good care of the self. This care of the self requires not only good physical habits, but good emotional habits.

Spiritual or "Positive" Emotions

Positive psychology in general has avoided spirituality and health. Yet spirituality and religious traditions are the primary contexts in which, for many people, positive emotions have their home. In other words, positive emotions flourish in authentic traditions of the Ontological Generality. Of course in distorted or false traditions, hatred and contempt can come to an unfortunate dominance.

Let me distinguish, for example, optimism from hope as "spiritual" positive emotion. This is more than semantic quibbling. Hope leans into the future with a deep trust that something good will come. It is so much more than mere optimism, which is mostly a present-tense gloss that lacks the depth of hope and that withers when tested. Hope has to go through trials and hard times, and so frequently is taught and conveyed through spiritualities and religions. If things are going smoothly for a while in life, optimism is good enough and we do not really need hope. Hope is about firmly asserting a purposeful energy in the face of adversity. We can be optimistic and content without having to hope. Hope involves more personal reflection and sheer courage than optimism, and it takes practice. We can speak of the strength to hope, but not of the strength to optimism. How do we help others to be hopeful in hard times? Hope is by nature a lot more irrational than rational. It is a passion for the possible, or even for impossible impossibilities. We live betwixt and between reality and our dreams, and the world needs dreamers. Hope leans forward or there is no hope at all. Hope is a practice, a habit, a virtue. Core goals and dreams require tenacity, and hope must be stubborn or there will be no miracles in our lives. Where does hope come from? From community or relationships, from within, from an inspiring role model, from helping others, from God? Let me suggest that for many people, hope is deeply ensconced in the Ontological Generality. It is hard to imagine Dr. Martin Luther King Jr., when he referred to the hope of the prophet Amos flowing from the mountains in his famous speech at the Washington Monument, using the word "optimism" instead.

Are spirituality and religion something like a shopping center for hope, love, gratitude, tranquility, joy, and the like? Given that the vast majority of peoples over the face of the earth place spiritualities and religions at the essential core of their lives, the ways in which these cultivate salutogenic positive emotions and help to displace negative ones achieves great significance. "Sin" has a lot to do with bitterness, with self-pitying, with ruminating, with vengeful thinking, with rage, with jealousy—in short, with all those tendencies that we see from childhood to old age in those whose emotional and spiritual energies are self-focused. The mutual love said to be experienced in the triadic structure of the Ontological Generality rightly manifested frees adherents from this brooding darkness.

Jonathan Edwards, in his classic *Treatise on the Religious Affections*,[28] did a splendid job of moving "religion" away from doctrine and toward the cultivation of a set of affections (emotional states) that he felt were established in a stable fashion at the interface of the human substrate and the Holy Spirit. Karl Rahner thought similarly.[29] How does the self-reported experience of the divine of godly love enliven and enhance a set of positive emotions that are also "primed" by the language games of religious communities? What have spirituality and religion to say about the connections among joy, self-giving love, hope, faith/trust, tranquility, and the like? In general, these emotional "gifts" come as a package.

Because many spiritualities and religions teach emotional self-control, especially over negative emotions (e.g., Buddhism and Christianity eschew anger and revenge), they can at their best free the agent from these burdens and their many noxious health effects. Of course, particular theological traditions matter—fear and anxiety before a vengeful God can be anything but healthy.

A Deeper Tranquility That Protects against Stress

The Ontological Generality creates a secure attachment for individuals who are otherwise existing in conditions of "separation anxiety," adrift from the "secure" bases that allow life to be navigated well, especially in its challenges. Attachment theorists believe that all of life can be understood as a journey in overcoming separation anxieties. As infants thrown into the world, we seek parental attachment, and as adults we seek marriages of genuine attachment and communities of secure giving and receiving of tender loving care. We seek this as patients in the relationships we have with physicians, nurses, and other health care staff. Theologically, the fact that across the globe the vast majority of people seek ultimate security in a relationship with a Higher Power indicates that because in the final analysis all secure attachments in a finite life span will wither, we need to feel loved by God, however defined, just as we need to feel loved by others. Human tranquility, serenity, and inner peace are to be found in the Ontological Generality, in a continuous *communitas* between God, self, and other. Might the vast majority of any associations between religion and health be the result of the fact that religions at their best provide the ultimate secure base in a temporal and frail mortal existence?

More Lasting Unions

Having just attended an ornate Hindu wedding ceremony in Connecticut, it occurs to me that perhaps religions benefit health mainly through encouraging more lasting unions through sacred ritual. In other words, the Ontological Generality creates a deeper and more lasting community between God, self, and other in the form of a God-centered marriage. It has been said that "the family that prays together stays together."

In her numerous studies, discussed in her book (with Maggie Gallagher), *The Case for Marriage*,[30] family sociologist Linda J. Waite makes the claim that married people live longer lives, have better health, and have happier and more successful children. This is especially true for married men. Waite makes the claim that wives encourage their husbands to take better care of themselves, while single men tend to be self-neglectful and engage in risky behaviors.

But such an explanation seems quite narrow. Nearly ten thousand men with high risk of heart disease were studied for over five years. Researchers from the Israeli Ischemic Heart Disease Study found that men were two times less likely to develop angina pectoris (chest pain from restriction of blood to the heart) if they felt they had a loving and supportive wife.[31] It may be the power of love rather than the mere insistence on getting to the doctor.

There is so much anxiety and ill health due to the instability of relationships in our modern culture. Marriages break up as soon as people realize that love requires patience and effort to be sustained. In the absence of that special form of the Ontological Generality that we refer to as sacred marriage, why make the effort?

Eschatological Visions of Social Status Inversion

Within the context of the Ontological Generality, we are all equal. This is not just equality with regard to the promise of eschatological equality and even prophetic reversal of status in the future. In the kingdom of God, the first will be last and the last will be first. But as a partly realized eschatology, the Ontological Generality in the form of a *communitas* of mutual love between God, self, and other has already radically eclipsed the social hierarchies of a distorted world of bullying, abuse, classism, racism, sexism, hypercognitivism, and the like. This suggests that especially for people of lower socioeconomic class, or who are in various ways oppressed in a world of exploitation and injustice, health benefits may be the result of the alleviation of low-status realities in the outside world through a spiritual-religious restoration of elevated status at least within the community of believers.

In the late 1960s, there began a famous study of men in the British civil service. Called the Whitehall Study, it was directed by Dr. Michael Marmot, director of the International Center for Health and Society at the University of London.[32] Data showed that rates of mortality—from all causes, and separate from other risk factors such as smoking or drinking—consistently and steadily decreased as men's civil service grade increased. Every single man had equal access to health care, but the men on the lowest rung of the ladder had three times the mortality rate as those in the highest rungs. A twenty-five-year follow-up showed that this connection persisted after retirement and even among men in their eighties. Marmot concluded that stress might be the hidden factor. The lower your status, the more stressed you feel, and you are treated with less respect and have less control over your life. So mortality is linked with hierarchical status, and rank matters.

Following this theory, it could be the case that because some spiritualities and religions offer a strong sense of equality, and even a reversal of social status in the kingdom of God, they may buffer mortality rates for those who are otherwise in low status positions in society. This could explain some of the findings of Dr. Neal M. Krause around urban African-American believers.[33]

Proximate Intercessory Prayer (PIP)

In the lived *communitas* of the Ontological Generality, we speak not of Distant Intercessory Prayer (DIP), which seems to have been shown to be ineffective.[34] Rather, we speak of Proximate Intercessory Prayer (PIP), with the intense social interaction, the frenzied loss of self in ecstatic community, and the laying on of hands.

Indeed, this is a case where the gold standard method of a double-blind randomized control study completely blinded researchers to the actual phenomenology of proximate healing (e.g., as captured in the portraits of Jesus in the New Testament, or by the work of a Heidi Baker in Mozambique). One must be there, in the community, to observe in detail the dynamics of PIP and measurable outcomes.

One variable in the study of religion and health, then, is the extent to which PIP is occurring in face-to-face interactions and perhaps showing effects by whatever mechanisms. The Ontological Generality may engage the energy of interpersonal healing with a passion and belief that is unmatched in any other context.

Avoiding Negative Behaviors

One assumes that members of any community grounded in the Ontological Generality will be living more idealistic life patterns of neighbor-love and benevolence. This alone should allow them to cultivate virtues rather than be susceptible to vices and their adverse effects. Pitirim Sorokin, in *The Ways and Power of Love* (1954), reported on his studies of mortality rates over the centuries.[35] He contrasted "aggressively egoistic" and "altruistic" people, designated as such by existing historical documentation. Sorokin found differences that he explained as follows:

> As to the comparative life spans of the aggressively egoistic and unaggressive altruistic human beings, the aggressive egoists and the leaders of aggressive social organizations have, as a general rule, a shorter life span than the saintly altruists and friendly good neighbors of the same countries and periods. The aggressive enmity, predatory ambition, strenuous competition, and insatiable pride of the egoistic individuals seems to adversely affect their physical, moral, and mental well-being in spite of a "conspicuous consumption," luxurious living, and full satisfaction of their biological needs. On the other hand, deep peace of mind, friendliness toward others, and devotion to God, Love, and Moral Duty seems to invigorate the health and prolong the life span of eminent and saintly altruists, in spite of their ascetic practices, lack of necessities, and other supposedly unhealthy conditions of their life and activity.
>
> This generalization is well supported by many sets of evidences: a) By the comparatively short life span of criminals, wretched kind of life they live, and by the highest rate of death by violence they die. b) By the data of psychosomatic medicine showing the negative influence of hateful, aggressive, and inimical emotions upon physical, moral, and mental health of individuals.[36]

Sorokin continued:

On the other hand, the life span of the saintly and eminent altruists has been far above that of their contemporaries. In spite of their asceticism, fastings, long vigils, and lack of many necessities they lived longer than their contemporaries, or even the monarchs and rulers of their time.

It is true that among the Christian Catholic saints the rate of death by violence was also exceptionally high during especially the first centuries of Christianity; all in all 37 percent of them died by violent death. . . . The vigorous vitality and comparatively long life of altruists are due to the beneficial effects of friendly emotions and altruistic disposition upon the health, longevity, and well-being of the individuals.[37]

He explained that while saints might die martyrs, those who did not have their lives cut short tended to live long lives, mainly due to positive emotions and altruistic dispositions. Aggressive egoists, by contrast, would more likely die younger by virtue of violence, and by negative emotions and their impact on health.

Sorokin, in *The Reconstruction of Humanity*, wrote that "love is one of the best therapies for curing many mental disorders; for the elimination of sorrow, loneliness, and unhappiness, for the mitigation of hatred and other antisocial tendencies; and above all for the ennoblement of human personality, for the release in man of his creative forces. . . ."[38]

The Encouragement of Altruism

Obviously, living under the sacred canopy of the Ontological Generality moves the self away from narcissism, solipsism, and sin. "I" becomes less important than "Thou." In a study that goes back to 1983, Larry Scherwitz and colleagues in California and Texas analyzed the speech patterns of 160 "Type A" personality subjects (i.e., always in a hurry, *easily moved to hostility and anger*, high levels of competitiveness and ambition) [emphasis added].[39] His findings showed that the incidence of heart attacks and other stress-related illnesses was highly correlated with the level of self-references (i.e., "I," "me," "my," "mine," or "myself") in the subject's speech during a structured interview. High numbers of self-references significantly correlated with heart disease, after controlling for age, blood pressure, and cholesterol. The researchers suggested that patients with more severe disease were more self-focused and less other-focused. They recommend that a healthier heart can result when a person is more giving, listens attentively when others talk, and does things that are unselfish. There is something about being self-obsessed or self-preoccupied that seems to add to stress and stress-induced physical illness.

Health benefits in religion may be most easily explained with reference to the de-selfing that encourages altruism[40] in the intersection of the vertical and horizontal dimensions of the Ontological Generality. Members of congregations typically engage in helping activities, such as working on a Habitat House project or feeding the hungry. Altruism, even beyond the boundaries of the *communitas* itself, is encouraged. If altruism within limits is salutogenic, then this may contribute considerably to any health and religion associations, at least where the love of neighbor is truly lived out. It is fairly well established that the horizontal axis has clear benefits. The year 2010 was an exciting year for research on health, happiness, and helping others. For starters, in the United Healthcare/Volunteer Match Do Good Live Well Study,[41] an online survey of a national sample of 4,582 American adults 18 years and older, these remarkable facts stand out:

- 41 percent of us volunteer an average of 100 hours per year (males: 39 percent, females: 42 percent; Caucasians: 42 percent, African-Americans: 39 percent, Hispanics: 38 percent) (69 percent of us donate money).
- 68 percent of volunteers agree that volunteering "has made me feel physically healthier," 92 percent that it "enriches my sense of purpose in life," 89 percent that it "has improved my sense of well-being," 73 percent that it "lowers my stress levels," 96 percent that it "makes people happier," 77 percent that it "improves emotional health," and 78 percent that it helps with recovery "from loss and disappointment."

- Volunteers have less trouble sleeping, less anxiety, less helplessness and hopelessness, better friendships and social networks, and a greater sense of control over chronic conditions.
- 25 percent volunteer through workplace, and 76 percent of them feel better about their employer as a result.

It would be difficult to identify any pill or vitamin with such a pronounced self-reported impact on so many lives. The survey was conducted by TNS (Taylor Nelson Sofres), the world's largest custom survey agency, from February 25–March 8, 2010.

Ralph Waldo Emerson, in a famous essay, wrote, "It is one of the most beautiful compensations of this life that no man can sincerely try to help another without helping himself. . . ."[42] The sixteenth-century Hindu poet Tulsidas, as translated by Mohandas K. Gandhi, wrote: "This and this alone is true religion—to serve others. This is sin above all other sin—to harm others. In service to others is happiness. In selfishness is misery and pain."[43] The ninth-century sage Shantideva wrote, "All the joy the world contains / Has come through wishing the happiness of others."[44] Proverbs 11:25 reads, "[T]hose who refresh others will themselves be refreshed" (NLT). Martin Buber described the moral transformation of shifting from "I-It" to "I-Thou," from a life centered on self as the center of the universe around whom, like the sun, all others revolve.[45] This "I" relates to others only as means to its own ends. But the spiritual and moral self of "I-Thou" discovers "the other as other," and relates to them in compassion and respect. There is still an "I," of course, but a deeper and better "I"; science now shows a happier and healthier "I" as well. Every major religion recommends the discovery of a deeper and more profound human nature, designated in various ways as the "true self." In Acts 20:35 (KJV), we find the words, "It is more blessed to give than to receive," and these echo down into the *Prayer of St. Francis*.[46] Now science says it is so.

THE FIRST CAVEAT

People Who Live Close to the Ontological Generality in This World Should Expect Some Unrest, Making "Health" Less Important than Defending the Generality Itself

Martyrs are not seeking health and longevity. This is not to suggest that they need to be condemned (e.g., King, Bonhoeffer). They are hopefully not seeking death, but it finds them and they accept it with courage. (Were they seeking destruction, we would be dealing with pathological masochism, which certainly does surface in the religious context.) Spirituality and religion should not be held hostage to health-related values in any absolute or primary sense. Penultimate values like health are very important, but they do not trump. Some things are more important than the preservation of health.

The greatest symbol of Unlimited Love is finally the cross. Jesus was nothing but pure love. He helped people as a teacher and a healer, and they began to gather around him. He found happiness in giving. But regrettably, he ran into a man who sought happiness in material possessions, such as Judas with his thirty pieces of silver, or the money changers on the Temple steps. He ran into people who were seeking their happiness in political or religious power. In the end, they tortured him. Good things do not always happen to good people. But the worst thing is never the last thing because in the end love wins under all conditions so long as we persist in abiding in it. This is what Jesus did, and he was the victor.

In general, people who live loving lives find life gratifying, meaningful, joyful, and hopeful. While they love others for their own sake, as a by-product they come to realize that in the giving of self lies the discovery of a deeper and more flourishing self. They will often find renewal and resilience in this gift-love when life gets challenging, as it can and does. Usually, they will find soul partners or deep friends who share their concerns and commitments as they journey in the path of love. Thus community forms around love. Love is not to be relegated to the arid, dry, lonely portrait of human suffering. There is buoyancy in love.

But sometimes love is utterly unappreciated, unacknowledged, and even mocked. People who love others and who have done no wrong may find themselves under attack, rejected, disrespected, and even hated. There is something about love that elicits fury, especially in those whose cynicism is threatened by love. The children of love do not seek their misery, nor should they ever. Such would be pathological. But sometimes suffering finds them, and they accept it. They wish it were not so, and yet they believe that if they continue to love to the very end, even unto death, there will be a mysterious new dawn that results, for their way of being in this world will leave its mark in ways great and small. Such unchanging love echoes in eternity.

Someone said that great visionary people have understood that doing the right thing will often cause some degree of misunderstanding and produce suffering. Other people expect goodness to be rewarded with trophies in one form or another. They sometimes lose faith and turn bitter when they encounter rejection and pain. But visionaries grow in faith during the desolate times. Other people perceive all pain as an evil waste. There is no greater visionary than the prophet who is responsible for the central chapters of Isaiah. This ancient seer saw that suffering could lead to healing and liberation.

We would prefer to think that loving servants of goodness would, after a long and healthy life, die peacefully in their beds and have all people speak well of them at their funerals. But this is too simplistic.

THE SECOND CAVEAT

Many Religious Traditions in Practice Distort the Ontological Generality and Become Horrifically Unhealthy

In a time when rage, fragmentation, and violence between the three Abrahamic faith traditions are so visible in our world, godly love faces major human impediments. Rescuing God's love and our world from the clutches and consequences of a demonic ethic glorifying separation, divisiveness, dominance, and cruelty is clearly no easy task. Perhaps the most hopeful resource for this rescue lies at the doctrinal core of each of the Abrahamic faith groups, regardless of the public messages of their leaders or proponents, at this or any other time, which might seem to argue quite the opposite.

This approach eschews the secular assumption that people in these traditions can or should take off their particular religious identities like clothes removed before a shower. The enlightened modernist may think in such terms, but most human beings around the world define themselves—their core identity, their values, their ultimate commitments—in terms of faiths that are absolutely essential. Thus, one must highlight the ideal of godly love for all people without exception through the windows of Abrahamic religious particularity. All three traditions also have theological warrants and casuistry for interreligious conflict. Which element dominates is dependent in large part on political, economic, and territorial scenarios.

At their best, each tradition has deepened the spirit of love in the world, from Damascus to the Holocaust rescuers under Trocme's guidance. How can we understand the profound goodness whereby people committed to love as inspired by their Abrahamic faith do deeds of radical goodness across group division, such as the Holocaust rescuers both Christian and Muslim?

Borrowing here from a list of questions drafted with Dr. Stephen Spector,[47] we might ask: What are the definitions and conceptual boundaries of divine love? Have these concepts evolved over time, in response to changing historical circumstances? What do sacred texts and holy people have to say? How do we access and manifest divine love? Are our love of God and our love of our fellow beings associated in some way? Are they inseparable (one joined to the other), conditional (one upon the other), hierarchical (one trumps the other), nested (one defined in terms of the other)? To what end does divine love influence the lives of individual human beings, the communion of believers, and the state of the world? Does divine love figure into discussions of personal or collective redemption or of eschatology? What are the forces arrayed against the apostles of divine love and what are the challenges to be overcome? What are the prospects of success? What are the major ways in which divine love has been distorted? When and where have distortions occurred in the past? Are they present and visible today? How can such distortions be avoided or corrected? Who are the great historic exemplars of divine love? How did they confront apostasy and distortions of divine love? Were they ultimately successful in their work of restoration? In what ways did they fail? Are the resources that they drew upon, internal to their faith tradition, available to believers in the present day? What can we learn from people in history and alive today who have truly demonstrated a cosmopolitan love for those in other traditions, many of whom have been deemed a threat by those who love just some small fragment of humanity?

Toward the end of his life, Sir John Templeton expressed reasonable ambivalence over these faith traditions because of continued conflict that he counted among the most destructive impediments to human progress. While he acknowledged the importance of tolerance between the Abrahamic faiths, he clearly saw tolerance as a rather minimalistic rung in a ladder of attitudinal progress rising upward to respect, trust, and, ultimately, to an authentic love between three faith traditions that share a common vision of a God of Unlimited Love. The theme of love between the adherents of the three Abrahamic faith traditions shaped Sir John's development of *humility theology*. Concerned with the potential of terrorism, he wrote a book entitled *Pure Unlimited Love: An Eternal Creative Force and Blessing Taught by All Religions*.[48] Sir John cited passages from the scriptures and sages of the three faiths (as well as from non-Abrahamic traditions) underscoring God's love for all people without exception. He emphasized "how little we know" about spiritual realities, and how much progress could be made if these religions would all aspire to take to heart and learn more about the one great aspiration that they hold in common—Unlimited Love.

Each of these faith traditions offers guidance on how we may grow toward identifying with a shared humanity rather than a mere fragment thereof, and on how each of us may come to see ourselves in the other; each tradition at its best seeks to shape a normative religious experience that guides its adherents toward recognition of a common humanity with believers on different spiritual paths. However, each tradition also contains restrictive elements that focus in a purely insular direction that may even devalue or demonize nonadherents. We do not assume that the Abrahamic traditions are identical in this regard. Yet each tradition can enunciate its commitment to Unlimited Love more vividly, and can be enhanced in the practice of such extensive love.

This theme of Unlimited Love is present in the sacred writings and the ideals of all the Abrahamic religions. To a significant degree, however, these great traditions have struggled to maintain their relevance, especially as secularism has partly eroded their confidence in the sacred.[49] The spiritual void left behind has found potent spiritualities anxious to fill the lacuna in a rising tide of fundamentalism, which has had a marked tendency toward an arrogant absolutism that demonizes and dehumanizes outsiders, redefining them as unworthy of God's love and grace.

Due to an emphasis on tribalistic elements in fundamentalist religion, over and above moral and ethical imperatives, norms of religious devotion may be observed to elicit harmful tendencies. The glorification of a favored identity (e.g., election, salvation) has made fundamentalism vulnerable to reifying the "otherness" of outsiders. This distorts the messages of love, unity, justice, compassion, kindness, and mercy that lie at the core of the great orthodox traditions, that serve to instill humility in religious believers, and that denote the essence of divine love.

Of course tribalism is not something that we question in its constructive form. The Abrahamic faith traditions are keenly cognizant of, and defined by, notions of peoplehood or nationhood. It does not serve to lay indirect blame for the crisis of our age at the feet of a generic tribalism. Common sense calls us to delineate the morally functional and dysfunctional, the good and the bad, in ritually bounded and supernaturally sanctioned communities. As Emile Durkheim observed, the members of tribal clans live in relationship with each other not primarily on account of shared kinship but due to mutual affiliation with totemic entities, including beliefs, that define the associative relations as sacred.[50] These tribalisms are functional—they serve to reaffirm and elevate the holiness of a people and thus ideally inspire and enable greater and more successful acts of communal and worldly service to exemplify that holiness.

By contrast, the tribalism that loses sight of a shared humanity is prone to moral dysfunction. *In extremis*, the tribal instinct as manifested within contemporary religious fundamentalists is not so much about affirming or elevating one's own holiness or sacred status for instrumental purposes as about judging and distancing oneself from otherness. The "other" is stigmatized, condemned, and avoided like the plague—and left to its reward in hell. In the contemporary world, systems of political-economy have been used by fundamentalists in attempts to marginalize and even criminalize the "other."

As I have written (again with Dr. Spector),[51] this runs counter to the founding principles of the aforementioned tribal religions. Instead of engendering withdrawal within our tribal borders or, alternatively, militant reaction, our contacts with the "other" can present challenges of learning and growth. We can come to see in our brothers and sisters distinct reflections of our mutual oneness that perhaps we cannot see through our own cultural lenses. Engaging the divine in our fellow beings thus presents opportunities to better recognize our own divine nature. *The enemy of progress is not tribalism* per se*, but rather the exploitation of tribalistic impulses dormant in respective religious traditions in order to marginalize, condemn, and attack other tribes, rather than to achieve Unlimited Love.*

Drawing here again on Sorokin's 1954 classic, *The Ways and Power of Love*, he developed a measure of love that involves five aspects. The first aspect of love is *intensity*. Low-intensity love involves minor actions, such as relinquishing a bus seat for another's comfort; high-intensity, by contrast, engages elevated levels of time, energy, and resources on the agent's part. Sorokin did not see the range of intensity as scalar—i.e., research cannot indicate "how many times greater a given intensity is than another,"[52] but it is possible to see "which intensity is really high and which low, and sometimes even to measure it."[53] The second aspect of love is *extensivity*: "The extensivity of love ranges from the zero point of love of oneself only, up to the love of all mankind, all living creatures, and the whole universe. Between the minimal and maximal degrees lies a vast scale of extensivities: love of one's own family, or a few friends, or love of the groups one belongs to—one's own clan, tribe, nationality, nation, religious, occupational, political, and other groups and associations."[54] Sorokin had immense respect for family love and friendships, but he clearly thought that people of great love lean outward toward all humanity without exception, and that truly great lovers inspire others to do the same. He understood human beings to have pronounced tendencies toward insular group love, and he argued that religion at its best moves agents beyond their insularities to humanity and even all life.

Sorokin was a scientific optimist, hoping that enhanced understanding might unlock the "enormous power of creative love"[55] to stop aggression and enmity and contribute to vitality and longevity,[56] cure mental illness, sustain creativity in the individual and in social movements, and provide the only sure foundation for ethical life. Sorokin's general law is as follows:

> *If unselfish love does not extend over the whole of mankind, if it is confined within one group—a given family, tribe, nation, race, religious denomination, political party, trade union, caste, social class or any part of humanity—such in-group altruism tends to generate an out-group antagonism.* And the more intense and exclusive the in-group solidarity of its members, the more unavoidable are the clashes between the group and the rest of humanity.[57]

Moreover, in-group exclusivism has "*killed more human beings and destroyed more cities and villages than all the epidemics, hurricanes, storms, floods, earthquakes, and volcanic eruptions taken together. It has brought upon mankind more suffering than any other catastrophe.*"[58] What is needed, argues Sorokin, is enhanced extensivity.

Sorokin placed his faith in science, as we do:

> Science can render an inestimable service to this task by inventory of the known and invention of the new effective techniques of altruistic ennoblement of individuals, social institutions, and culture. Our enormous ignorance of love's properties, of the efficient ways of its production, accumula-

tion, and distribution, of the efficacious ways of moral transformation has been stressed many times in this work.[59]

CONCLUSIONS

Let us completely rebuild the field of religion and health without the agenda of proving that "religion is good for health." Honesty and objectivity require greater nuance. To date, the field has been too easy on itself, and has suffered the consequences. We need something more nuanced. Part of the problem is the inevitable result of a field where serious dialogue between theologians and researchers has never occurred at the deepest level, nor engaged the best theological minds. I have tried to suggest how a theological anthropology, the Ontological Generality, can help to at least open up the interpretive complexity of any association between religion and health. I have also suggested that research needs to focus on the specifics of those traditions that are salutogenic, and be clear in asserting that many religious and spiritual traditions are notably unhealthy—as when the Jain mystic starves himself to death rather than take the chance of injecting anything living, including such things as bacteria or yeast.

The field is suffering because few scholars in the field are thinking out of the box, or offering new creative visions. Part of the problem is that major theological minds and comparative religion scholars should be front and center, but the field has done a poor job to date of drawing in these more conceptual thinkers. High-level scientific researchers should be in significant and sustained dialogue with these different sorts of minds, for otherwise they tend not to ask new and better questions. Instead, they get stuck in what they know—the technocracy of method. Social science is inherently reductive. Technocrats have overwhelmed visionary minds, and yet the two need each other in a creative synergy that has not happened. Thus, there has been an unnecessary and counterproductive divide between the researchers and the theologians. The former are too simple with their numbers and interpretations, while the latter have wished no association with such medicalization of religion.

The field needs a rebirth. This will need to involve high-level religious scholars, positive psychologists, theologians, experts in preventive and behavioral medicine, global health sociologists of religion, cultural anthropologists who study health-related rites of passage, medical/ health historians, researchers who have studied mortality and prolongevity in relation to many variables (optimism, happiness, altruism, curiosity, social capital, lasting marriages, faith, religion, spirituality, creativity, social status, race and class, ethnicity), and many others who are ready for an integrative maturity. We need researchers who have a genuine interest in dialogue with religious thinkers, and vice versa. Theology and *praxis* in faith community must be much more involved and shaped, which means that leading academics and clergy (including members from all Abrahamic faiths) must be engaged seriously. We need to consider visionary goals that only come from melding deep science, deep religious thought, deep integration, deep strategy, and leadership that does not accept the silos of the past.

NOTES

1. Jeff Levin, "'And Let Us Make Us a Name': Reflections on the Future of the Religion and Health Field," *Journal of Religion and Health* 48 (2009): 125–45, quotation on 129.
2. Søren Kierkegaard, *The Concept of Anxiety: A Simple Psychologically Orienting Deliberation on the Dogmatic Issue of Hereditary Sin* [1844], ed. and trans. Reider Thomte with Albert A. Anderson (Princeton, NJ: Princeton University Press, 1980).
3. Matthew 22:37–40 (AKJV).
4. David Brooks, "Bill Wilson's Gospel," *New York Times*, June 28, 2010, accessed at http://www.nytimes.com/2010/06/29/opinion/29brooks.html.
5. *Alcoholics Anonymous: The Story of How Many Thousands of Men and Women Have Recovered from Alcoholism* [1939], 4th ed. (New York: Alcoholics Anonymous World Services, 2001).
6. Ibid., xxv.
7. Ibid., xxvi.
8. Ibid., 201.
9. Ibid., 62.
10. Ibid., 63.
11. Ibid.
12. Ibid., 20.
13. Ibid., 18.
14. Ibid., 89.
15. Ibid., 62.
16. Ibid.
17. Ibid., 60.
18. Ibid., 20.
19. Ibid., 70.
20. Ibid., 94.
21. Ibid., 93.
22. Ibid., 100.

23. Maria E. Pagano, Karen B. Friend, J. Scott Tonigan, and Robert L. Stout, "Helping Other Alcoholics in Alcoholics Anonymous and Drinking Outcomes: Findings from Project MATCH," *Journal of Studies on Alcohol* 65 (2004): 766–73.

24. Maria E. Pagano, Brie B. Zeltner, Jihad Jaber, Stephen G. Post, William H. Zywiak, and Robert L. Stout, "Helping Others and Long-term Sobriety: Who Should I Help to Stay Sober?" *Alcohol Treatment Quarterly* 27 (2009): 38–50.

25. Pagano et al., "Helping Other Alcoholics in Alcoholics Anonymous and Drinking Outcomes."

26. Ibid., 766.

27. Pagano et al., "Helping Others and Long-term Sobriety."

28. Jonathan Edwards, *Treatise on the Religious Affections* [1746] (New Haven, CT: Yale University Press, 1959).

29. See Karl Rahner, "Experience of Self and Experience of God" [1971], in *Karl Rahner: Theologian of the Graced Search for Meaning*, ed. Geoffrey B. Kelly (Minneapolis: Fortress Press, 1992), 172–83.

30. Linda J. Waite and Maggie Gallagher, *The Case for Marriage: Why Married People Are Happier, Healthier, and Better Off Financially* (New York: Broadway Books, 2000).

31. Jack H. Medalie and Uri Goldbourt, "Angina Pectoris among 10,000 Men. II. Psychosocial and Other Risk Factors as Evidenced by a Multivariate Analysis of a Five Year Incidence Study," *American Journal of Medicine* 60 (1976): 910–21.

32. Michael Marmot, *The Status Syndrome: How Social Standing Affects Our Health and Longevity* (New York: Henry Holt, 2005).

33. See studies cited throughout Neal M. Krause, *Aging in the Church: How Social Relationships Affect Health* (West Conshohocken, PA: Templeton Foundation Press, 2008).

34. Herbert Benson, Jeffery A. Dusek, Jane B. Sherwood, Peter Lam, Charles F. Bethea, William Carpenter, Sidney Levitsky, Peter C. Hill, Donald W. Clem, Manoj K. Jain, David Drumel, Stephen L. Kopecky, Paul S. Mueller, Dean Marek, Sue Rollins, and Patricia L. Hibberd, "Study of the Therapeutic Effects of Intercessory Prayer (STEP) in Cardiac Bypass Patients: A Multicenter Randomized Trial of Uncertainty and Certainty of Receiving Intercessory Prayer," *American Heart Journal* 151 (2006): 934–42.

35. Pitirim A. Sorokin, *The Ways and Power of Love: Types, Factors, and Techniques of Moral Transformation* [1954], with an "Introduction" by Stephen G. Post (Philadelphia, PA: Templeton Press, 2002).

36. Ibid., 475.

37. Ibid., 476.

38. Pitirim A. Sorokin, *The Reconstruction of Humanity* (Boston: Beacon Press, 1948), 225.

39. Larry Scherwitz, Robert McKelvain, Carol Laman, John Patterson, Laverne Dutton, Solomon Yusim, Jerry Lester, Irvin Kraft, Donald Rochelle, and Robert Leachman,

"Type A Behavior, Self-Involvement, and Coronary Atherosclerosis," *Psychosomatic Medicine* 45 (1983): 47–57.

40. Stephen G. Post, ed., *Altruism and Health: Perspectives From Empirical Research* (New York: Oxford University Press, 2007).

41. "Volunteer for Healthier Communities" (2001), accessed at http://www.dogoodlivewell.org/UnitedHealthcase-VolunteerMatch-DoGoodLiveWell-Survey.pdf.

42. Quotation attributed to Ralph Waldo Emerson, cited in Lilian Eichler Watson, comp., *Light from Many Lamps* (New York: Fireside, 1951), 168.

43. Quotation attributed to Tulsidas, cited in Stephen G. Post, "It's Good To Be Good: 2011 Fifth Annual Scientific Report on Health, Happiness and Helping Others," *International Journal of Person Centered Medicine* 1 (2001), accessed at http://www.ijpcm.org/index.php/IJPCM/article/view/154.

44. Shantideva, *The Way of the Boddhisattva (Bodhicharyāvatāra)* [c. 700], rev. ed., trans Padmakara Translation Group (Boston: Shambhala, 2006), 127 (8.29).

45. Martin Buber, *I and Thou*, trans. Walter Kauffman (New York: Charles Scribner's Sons, 1970).

46. For a history of the *Prayer of St. Francis* [c. thirteenth century], see Christian Renoux, *La Prière pour la Paix Attribuée à Saint François, une Énigme à Résoudre* (Paris: Editions Franciscaines, 2001).

47. Stephen G. Post and Stephen Spector, unpublished grant proposal, 2009.

48. John Marks Templeton, *Pure Unlimited Love: An Eternal Creative Force and Blessing Taught by All Religions* (Philadelphia, PA: Templeton Press, 2000).

49. This discussion of fundamentalism, tribalism, and Durkheim revisits themes discussed in Jeff Levin and Stephen G. Post, eds., *Divine Love: Perspectives from the World's Religious Traditions* (West Conshohocken, PA: Templeton Press, 2010), especially Jeff Levin, "Introduction: Divine Love in the World's Religious Traditions," 3–22.

50. Emile Durkheim, *The Elementary Forms of Religious Life*, trans. Joseph Ward Swain (1912; repr. New York: The Free Press, 1915).

51. Post and Spector.

52. Sorokin, *The Ways and Power of Love*, 15.

53. Ibid.

54. Ibid., 16.

55. Ibid., 48.

56. Ibid., 60–61.

57. Ibid., 459; italics in original.

58. Ibid., 461.

59. Ibid., 477.

JOHN SWINTON

9. FROM HEALTH TO *SHALOM*

Why the Religion and Health Debate Needs Jesus

One of the things that troubles me about the various debates that go on around the issue of whether or not religion is good for your health is the absence of Jesus.[1] As I read through the wide and diverse literature on religion and health, rarely do I hear the name of Jesus. Much is written about a generic category described as "religion," which it seems can be good for a person's physiological and psychological health, but when it comes to the specifics of religion, religious beliefs, and the referent of the religious system—God—there seems to be a strange silence. It is true that some are pushing us to reflect on the importance of the particularities of beliefs for health,[2] but even then it is the belief, rather than the referent of the beliefs, that seems to be the primary focus of interest. It seems that it is what we believe *about* Jesus (or any other divine figure) that is important rather than what we know Jesus himself.

As one reads through the literature that claims to reflect on the ways in which religion and religious traditions can enable human well-being, I as a participant in religion would expect to encounter rich, interdisciplinary reflections on the deep theological meanings of illness and the implications of such meanings for health and discipleship. Instead what we discover are thin, generic, and nondenominational definitions of religion that are correlated with particular physiological or psychological changes that can be observed and measured in participants. So, for example, Harold Koenig in his important collection of data relating to the positive correlation of religion with mental health, *The Handbook of Religion and Mental Health,* offers an understanding of religion in these terms:

> It is important to note the following: (a) A traditional, broad definition of religion is used here, one that includes both personal-spiritual and institutional expressions of faith; and (b) this evaluation of the effects of religion on the coping process is not based on the ultimate truth of any religious creed. Scientists cannot determine whether there is a God, whether people really experience miracles, or the ultimate truth of religious teachings. What can be evaluated scientifically is whether religious methods of coping affect adjustment to difficult negative life circumstances and if so how.[3]

Putting aside for a moment the question of precisely what "a traditional, broad definition of religion" might actually look like and whose tradition might form its basis, it is not difficult to see some problems with this way of looking at religion. First, such a perspective reduces religion to nothing more than a set of beliefs and behaviors that may or may not help a person physically or psychologically. Religion is stripped of its central concern with ultimate truth and is presented as simply another mode of human behavior that scientists can look at and measure in exactly the same ways as they look at and measure any other phenomenon. It makes little difference whether Jesus is real, as long as the effects of believing in him can be measured. There may be some methodological sense in reducing religion to certain observable behaviors and changes and excluding issues of "ultimate truth." However, bearing in mind that issues of ultimate truth are the very reason that most religions exist, would such an understanding of religion be even vaguely recognizable to participants within particular traditions? The dissonance of such a position is brought out nicely by Billy Sunday's observation that "going to church on Sunday does not make you a Christian any more than going into a garage makes you an automobile!"[4] Likewise, believing that one can define religion by looking only at behaviors and psychological processes is like looking at a picture of a summer's day in Boston and imagining that one really now knows what it is like to experience a summer's day in Boston!

Second, such an understanding of religion seems to assume that the scientific task does not involve making claims about ultimate truth. The scientific task in relation to religion, it is presumed, is simply to adopt a neutral stand wherein the particular health benefits of specific beliefs and behaviors can be observed and measured effectively and accurately. Of course, the irony of claiming that science cannot discern the ultimate truth of religious teachings is that in order to propose this one must, presumably, know the nature of ultimate truth. However, as Job's question correctly highlights, no one can know the depths of God: "Can you fathom the mysteries of God? Can you probe the limits of the Almighty?"[5] We therefore have little idea as to whether science can or cannot discern the nature of ultimate truth. So why exclude it? Why separate the theological task from the practical outworking of religion when in fact the practical outworking may be deeply significant for our understanding of the nature of ultimate truth? Why begin from a philosophical and theological position of dualism and materialism when a theologically informed wholism might more accurately reflect the phenomenon being observed? Excluding issues of ultimate truth is far from a neutral move.

Third, the suggestion that scientists cannot determine whether there is a God is highly problematic even if it may be true. As we will see, in practice, scientists frequently make implicit and explicit statements about the nature of God. So whilst it is true to state that the existence of God cannot be proved by science, as I will try to show in this chapter, scientists clearly have opinions and perspectives on God and how God functions in the world that deeply influence the way in which they go about the task of researching religion and health. Why else would one assume that one can exclude questions about God and ultimate truth from the scientific exploration of religion and health? Is this not a deep theological statement?

Finally, as a Christian and a theologian, it is difficult to see in what sense such a definition in any way represents or encapsulates the nature of my faith tradition, which is *wholly* based on the ultimate truth of its religious creed and *wholly* based on the ultimate truth of its Scriptures and traditions. In what sense could a scientist claim to be looking at my religion when the very reason for its existence becomes the criteria for its exclusion from the scientific venture? As a Christian and a disciple of Jesus, it makes little sense to suggest that the truth of my beliefs are epiphenomenal to the practices that emerge from them. The idea that one can set aside issues of ultimate truth in order to look at the behaviors that emerge from believing in ultimate truth is a bit like a person's thumb saying, "If you look at me, you will be able to understand the whole of the body!" If the reply is that the religion and health research is not intended to look at the whole of religion, but only those parts that can be measured in relation to health and well-being without their theological overlay, we end up in exactly the same position: "Look at me! I'm a thumb!! You don't have to look at the whole body to know that thumbs are good for you." But, of course, important as the functions of thumbs are, they are not the whole of the body, nor can looking at them enable one to see the whole of the body. A body cannot find its definition in its thumbs. The healthy function of the thumb only makes proper sense in the context of the *telos* of the body.[6] Likewise, as I will argue below, the proper understanding of any health benefits that might be related to participation in religion only makes sense within the context of the whole of a religious system, including those fundamental issues of ultimate truth that make religion religion.

The intention of this chapter is to open up some critical questions that seek to examine precisely what scientific research into the relationship between religion and health thinks it is doing and whether such intentions are (a) plausible, and (b) theologically appropriate. I will suggest that there are serious questions to be asked on both points, but that there may also be ways forward for constructive dialogue.

RELIGION AND HEALTH: WHAT EXACTLY ARE WE LOOKING AT?

Perhaps the first thing to notice as we approach the field of religion and health is how vague the basic concepts actually are. The suggestion that religion is good for your health is alluring, but precisely what either of these terms actually means is remarkably unclear. There is no single thing called "religion." The term represents a diversity of beliefs, cultures, traditions, and practices. Even within so-called traditional religions, there is a huge variety of beliefs from liberal, to conservative, to charismatic, to fundamentalist, and a variety of different practices and ways of doing community. This diversity explains why it is that researchers often like to offer a basic definition of the understanding of religion that underpins their research at the beginning of their research reports. It is therefore important to begin by noting that such "working definitions" have been constructed by the researcher for the purposes of her study. They may or may not resonate with religious adherents, but that is not their point. The definitions are constructed in order that certain things can be included and other aspects excluded. The general intention seems to be to develop ways of looking at religion that turn it into a global concept, the general features of which can be examined and measured according to global indices across contexts.

The problem with this approach is that, except at a very basic level, religion is not a global concept. It is a complex and fragmented series of perspectives that contain as many unique and nonrepeatable aspects as they do generalizable concepts. In order to generalize, certain common features need to be melded together in a way that will enable the methods of science to measure and make sense of the impact of certain practices. In this way religion is reduced to sets of behaviors, values, and ways of being together in order that correlations can be found that match our perceptions of what is or is not a healthy side effect of religion. That being so, it is quite clear that we often make decisions and assumptions about the nature of religion that are much more pragmatic than scientific and more practical than spiritual.

If we were researching the effects of something like penicillin, this might not be a problem. But *religion is not medicine*. Often all that is being talked about is the simple fact that people like company and that community can be a good thing.[7] You do not need to believe anything in particular; you just need to be with friends. People believe certain things that are helpful when they are troubled and other things that are not so helpful. The fact that what they believe in has religious connotations is epiphenomenal to its measurable impact on scales of health. My point is not that such observations and effects are unhelpful or unimportant; it is just that they are deeply incomplete and inadequate in representing the nature of religion. If, for pragmatic reasons, religion is reduced to a global concept that can be measured according to global indices, then the fact that I love Jesus may be helpful to me, but it means nothing to those who are measuring me. This is deeply unsatisfactory for me as a believer, but surely it cannot be helpful scientifically either. If that which is being measured is not really what the scientist thinks it is, how can she be sure what she is measuring?

Health

Religion is a complicated concept. But so also is health. If we are claiming that religion is good for our health, we need to be clear about what health is. There are a number of different models of health that can be chosen to make sense of human experience. In Figure 9.1, David Seedhouse offers a useful overview of some of the key theories of health.

Seedhouse's diagram indicates that there are a wide range of ways in which health can be defined and understood.[8] It seems quite clear that the model of health that underpins the general ethos of the religion and health literature is the approach of medical science, which runs in tandem with Seedhouse's model of "health as a commodity" The other models of health may be of relevance, but it is this model that seems to lend itself most easily to the scientific investigation of religion and health. That might not immediately strike people as a problem. One might ask, "How else can science function?" However, there are significant issues with this approach. Think of it in this way.

FIGURE 9.1. Theories of Health.

From David Seedhouse, *Health: The Foundations for Achievement* (London: Wiley-Blackwell, 2001), 28.

THEORIES OF HEALTH

The theory that health is an ideal state:
- A 'Socratic' goal of perfect well-being in every respect
- An end in itself
- Disease, illness, handicap, and social problems must be absent

The theory that health is the physical and mental fitness to do socialised daily tasks (i.e. to function normally in a person's own society):
- A means towards the end of normal social functioning
- All disabling disease, illness, and handicap must be absent

The theory that health is a commodity which can be bought or given:
- The rational which lies behind medical theory and practice
- Usually an end for the provider, a means for the receiver
- Health is lost in the presence of disease, illness, pain, malady. It must be restored piecemeal.

A group of theories which hold that health is a personal strength or ability – either physical, metaphysical, or intellectual
- These strengths and abilities are not commodities which can be given or purchased. Nor are they ideal states. They are developed as personal tasks. They can be lost. They can be encouraged.

APPROACHES DESIGNED TO INCREASE HEALTH

The sociological approach
- Concerned with a range of factors which influence health—for good or bad. Works to describe unequal distribution of disease and illness, and the unequal use of the Health Service by different sections of the community. Tries to explain the causes of these inequalities in terms of socio-economic, political, personal, environmental, biological, and change factors.
- Its findings are used to provoke changes in society.

The approach of medical science
- Emphasis on clinics, hospitals, biology, statistics, and measurement of conditions against normal standards.
- The causes of disease and the effects of drugs and surgical techniques are researched to increase understanding and to allow preventive, curative, and educational measures.

The humanist approach
- Regards as a positive goal to be achieved personally. Disease, illness, and other problems can coexist with health
- Recognises that people are complex wholes living within, and permanently influenced by, a constantly changing world. Recognises that there are interconnections between the physical, the spiritual, and the intellectual.

COMMON FACTOR

In general, the provision of the conditions necessary for the achievement of some biological and chosen potentials, and some conditions which enable people to work towards the achievement of other biological and chosen potentials is the goal of all approaches. Much of the provision of suitable conditions is achieved by the removal of obstacles.

Why is it that data such as the following should be considered indicators of the benefits of religion for *health*?:

Religion has been found to:

- Extend life expectancy.[9]
- Lower blood pressure.[10]
- Lower rates of death from coronary artery disease.[11]
- Reduce anxiety.[12]
- Alleviate depression.[13]
- Reduce levels of pain in cancer sufferers.[14]
- Reduce mortality among those who attend church and worship services.[15]
- Reduce mortality after cardiac surgery.[16]

Now it might seem obvious to the reader that these things are indicators of health. However, such "obviousness" may simply reflect the deep ways in which the approach of medical science is powerful and embedded within our worldviews and our constructions of health and illness. It is almost impossible to think of health or illness without first thinking about medicine. Bearing in mind the wide diversity of ways in which we *could* define health and the diversity of ways in which we deal with illness, most of which do not involve medicine, this simple observation is quite telling. It is not that the benefits to our bodies and minds of participating in religion are undesirable. My point is simply that equating any of these side effects of religion with "health" reflects a quite specific understanding of what the researcher thinks health is. Such an understanding emerges from a combination of a basic method that focuses on measuring things and an approach drawn from medical science that conceives of health primarily as the absence of some form of pathological process or experience. But why do those working within the field of religion and health choose this model of health rather than the others?

FOUR TENSIONS WITHIN CURRENT APPROACHES TO RESEARCHING RELIGION AND HEALTH

In seeking an answer to this question, it will be helpful to focus on four tensions within current approaches to researching religion and health. In drawing out these tensions, the reasons for my initial observation about the lack of Jesus in the research will become clear. We might outline these tensions under four headings:

1. A positivistic mood of enquiry.
2. Implicit theological assumptions within scientific approaches.
3. The genericization of religion.
4. A primary dependence on measurement.

A Positivistic Mood of Enquiry

The general tenor of the conversations that emerge from the exploration of religion and health tend to be positivistic in tone. Positivism can be understood as a "philosophical system that holds that every rationally justifiable assertion can be scientifically verified or is capable of logical or mathematical proof."[17]

Within such an approach, issues of metaphysics, theology, or God become highly problematic. They represent a quite different epistemology. Positivism has had a profound impact on the way in which health services have been developed, research has been carried out, and strategies for care have been constructed, tested, and thought through. In terms of the religion and health research agenda, my suggestion is not so much that researchers embrace positivism as a formal philosophy. It is more that, as Gregory Baum puts it,[18] there is a "positivistic mood" that surrounds the research that allows people to see some things but also prevents them from seeing other important things. To be acceptable as evidence, we need to be able to *see* or *measure* the phenomenon at hand. Theology and the ultimate reality of spiritual experience may well be helpful for people at a personal, psychological level, but such faith cannot be measured and therefore cannot be proven via the methods of science. Faith, as the writer to the Hebrews puts it, is being sure of what you hope for and certain of what you cannot see.[19] Faith-based evidence makes little sense within a context that assumes the primacy of positivism as the gateway to authentic knowledge. This is a rather odd position when, as will become clear, some form of faith underpins the approaches of both religion and science.

What do we really see when we look?

Underpinning this positivistic mood is a quite particular philosophical position: *empiricism.* For those who adhere to this philosophy, Brent Slife informs us:

> The primary authority for truth lies in observation or sensory experience. This movement grew out of the recognition that logic and rationality—rationalism—are only as valid as their initial premises, and that premises cannot themselves be logically derived. Empiricists held that valid premises come from valid observations of the world.[20]

Within this perspective, only that which falls upon the retina of the eye can be considered factual in terms of a form of truth that is public and verifiable, as opposed to opinion or experience that is personal and therefore not publicly verifiable.

Within an empirically oriented research context, the benefits of religion have to be *seen* and *measured* if they are to be considered authentic (hence the exclusion of the ultimate truth of beliefs). This of course is where things become tricky. God can neither be seen nor measured. In order to "measure the spiritual" (which is by definition intangible and ethereal), it is necessary to *operatioanalize* it, that is, to *translate* it into physical terms that are measurable and quantifiable. This translation can be into concepts or into numbers, but it always involves a movement from the intangibility of spirituality and spiritual experience into some form of physical, observable data. The problem is that when religion is translated solely into the empirical, the resulting findings may have little to do with the original ideas that were present before translation, particularly if the ideas conflict with the philosophy and epistemology of the research method in the first place. When this happens rather strange things begin to occur.

For example, we find scientists claiming that prayer "doesn't work" because it doesn't provide results that are measurable according to the criteria laid down by the researchers.[21] Likewise, we find scientists claiming that prayer *does* work based on the same criteria.[22] Both conclusions are quite interesting, but as a Christian I am not at all convinced that my belief in prayer or its perceived efficacy is determined by the success or otherwise of randomized control trials! In my reading of the Scriptures, I see no indication that God should be tested in this way. Actually quite the opposite seems to be the case: "Jesus answered, 'It says: "Do not put the Lord your God to the test."'"[23]

But beyond this obvious theological problem, there is a deeper philosophical problem lurking behind the approach of empiricism. Empiricism is a *philosophical* position. It is necessary to adhere to the philosophical belief before one can assume that empiricism is the most authentic way to gain knowledge. However, *there is no empirical evidence for empiricism*! The assumption that all that there is is what one can see is simply a statement of faith based on particular philosophical assumptions (a combination of philosophical materialism and empiricism) about the nature of the world—philosophical assumptions that cannot be proven by the philosophy's own criteria. A statement such as "there is no evidence for the efficacy prayer" is a statement of faith based on certain methodological, epistemological, and probably cosmological presuppositions about the way the world is and what can and cannot be used as criteria for truth. It seems that faith—being sure of what you hope for and certain of what you cannot see—is not something that is the sole domain of religious people.

Implicit Theological Assumptions

It is interesting to note that although there appears to be an inherent division between religious faith and the empirical demands of science, a deeper reflection reveals that there is in fact a good deal of theology going on within the scientific exploration of religion and health. The strange thing is that, even for scientists who claim to have some form of religious commitment, there appears to be a gap between what they believe about God and how they function within the context of a worshipping community and the ways in which they function within the research community. For example, if one looks at the methods and results sections of the research on religion and health, certain key questions rarely if ever appear:

- Did the researcher pray about which method should be used?
- Did she ask God for guidance as she analyzed her data?
- Did the researcher reflect on God as part of her analysis?
- Did she assume her work was being carried out within *Creation* or a neutral context: "the world"?

It may of course be that all of these questions are answered in the affirmative by religiously oriented scientists. But why are they not written about? Why are such questions not central to the whole religion and health enterprise?

Methodological Deism?

The literature is speckled with scientists and psychologists stating that it is not their task to comment on the authenticity of belief systems, the implication being that the reality or unreality of religious systems makes no real difference to the scientific enterprise. This seems to be a rather odd position. Is the suggestion that one can reduce religious systems and beliefs to the measurement of particular behaviors and physiological changes not already a strong theological statement? Surely to suggest that the bodies of participants within particular religious systems can be measured and understood without any direct reference to God tells one something quite precise about how the researcher views God? Peter Berger has suggested that the term *methodological atheism* be used to describe theologians and historians who study religion as a human creation without declaring whether individual religious beliefs are actually true.[24] It might be unfair to apply this term to religious researchers exploring the relationship between religion and health. However, whilst atheism may be too strong a term, there is clearly a form of *methodological deism* at work: Slife describes methodological deism thus:

Natural science methods never require that investigators pray (or generally consult God or revelation) before designing or conducting a study. This requirement is omitted because God's current activities are presumed to be irrelevant to designing and conducting an effective investigation (though God's created order might be considered relevant to the results of the investigation).[25]

Active recognition of the present actions of God would be methodologically inappropriate as such actions cannot be seen according to the dual lenses of positivism and empiricism. God as creator thus becomes a secondary, unmeasurable aspect of the religion-health equation that can have little real value to the scientific enterprise other than as background noise to the more general exploration of health as it is defined by the researcher. Berger talks about the "flattening out" of religion that emerges from the scientific gaze:

> The functional approach to religion, whatever the original theoretical intention of its authors, serves to provide quasiscientific legitimations of a secularized world view. . . . The specificity of the religious phenomenon is avoided by equating it with other phenomenon. The religious phenomenon is "flattened out." Finally it is no longer perceived. Religion is absorbed into a night in which all cats are grey. The greyness is the secularised view of reality in which any manifestation of transcendence are . . . meaningless, and *therefore* can only be dealt with in terms of social or psychological functions that can be understood without reference to transcendence.[26]

It is strange to think that a Christian researcher might be comfortable with a flat Jesus whose followers are reduced to what they do, rather than who they do what they do for.

The Genericization of Religion

All of this helps to explain the reasons for the general tendency toward the genericization of religion that I have discussed previously. By the term *genericization*, I mean the assumption that religion can be flattened out in such a way as to strip it of its particularities in order to find common sets of experiences that are generalizable across religious boundaries. Such genericization is apparent in the language we use around issues of religion and health: "Religion is good for your health"; "the relationship between religion and health"; and so forth. Religion thus finds its definition not in God, but in human actions and responses. This seems like a curious mode of anthropocentrism or perhaps even idolatry wherein the focus is wholly on the creature to the exclusion of those features of religion that point toward the creator. Such genericization may be methodologically necessary in terms of the goals of the research and the way that health is defined, but it is clearly theologically highly problematic. The flattening out and genericization of religion might have some benefits in terms of measuring the effects of religion, but there is a real price to pay.

A Primary Dependence on Measurement

We have already seen the ways in which measurement has become important and some of the reasons for such an emphasis. Here it will be enough to note that whether religion is perceived as good for your health or otherwise depends on the criteria of health, well-being, and the understanding of "the good life" that the researcher has in mind and the specific measures that she chooses to use to assess it. The vast majority of research into the efficacy of religion for health has focused on psychological, social, or physical health criteria. However, the primary criterion of health for religious believers is spiritual. Health and well-being within religious traditions is very often not gauged by the *absence* of illness or distress, but by the *presence* of God-in-relationship. It is this observation that brings us back to my opening comments relating to the absence of Jesus from the religion and health conversations. For people who adhere to other or no religious traditions, the absence of Jesus makes little difference. Indeed, for the reasons outlined previously, the *presence* of Jesus makes little methodological or epistemological sense. However, things are necessarily different for Christians who wish to explore the relationship between *Christianity* and health. The reason for this is quite simple: within this tradition *Jesus is health*.

This is a critical observation that requires some explanation. As I have suggested, health (like religion) has many dimensions and multiple definitions. For the most part the understanding of health that guides the religion and health research emerges from the perspective of medical science. There is nothing wrong with that in itself, as long as such understandings are perceived in their proper context of creation, salvation, and redemption. Problems arise for Christians when our understandings of health are shorn from this context and placed in a revised framework that claims that it is possible to understand and measure the health of creatures without direct reference to the creator or the significance of creation.

From Health to Shalom

It is probably not coincidental that the Bible has no word for health as we have come to use the term within medical science. The closest approximation to contemporary understandings of health is the Hebrew word *shalom* (*Salôm*), which occurs 250 times in the Hebrew Bible. The basic meaning of the word *shalom* is peace. This peace encompasses physical and psychological health, but it is not defined by it. The root meaning of the word *shalom* is *wholeness, completeness,* and *well-being.*[27] *Shalom* is therefore a relational term that has primarily to do with a restoration of relationships, but more specifically the restoration of human beings with God. To be at peace—to be healthy—is to be in right relationship with God. Such relationship is not dependent on physical or psychological well-being, although such things obviously contribute to the experience of *shalom*. *Shalom* has several subsidiary meanings that emerge from this primary relational intention:

- security
- friendship
- prosperity
- justice
- righteousness
- salvation.[28]

These meanings flow from the primary relationship that God has with human beings. When that relationship is right, these other things occur naturally. When that relationship is broken, the subsidiary meanings are lost.

Within this understanding of human well-being, physical and psychological health is important. Hebraic anthropology perceives human beings as deeply interrelated creatures who have no separation between body and soul. To use Wheeler Robinson's phrase, the human is "an animated body, and not an incarnated soul."[29] Human bodily existence (which includes health as defined by medical science) is profoundly important to God, a fact marked out decisively within the incarnation and in particular the healing ministry of Jesus. However, such health is important only as it contributes to the ongoing implementation of God's *shalom*. The fact that religion is good for your medical health only has significance if one recognizes what such health is *for*: the glory of God.[30] Bodies matter, but only as they orient people toward the true source of health: Jesus.

Shalom Is a Person

Theologically then, health is not a biomedical category, it is a theological statement. More than that, health is not something you have or develop in your own strength by participating or not participating in religious ceremonies or practices. Health (*shalom*) is a gift of God's self to human beings. In the Hebrew Bible it is Yahweh Himself who is the source and giver of *shalom*. Wilkinson observes:

> One of the covenant names for God which Gideon used when he built his altar to the Lord at Oprah was Yahweh-*shalom*, the Lord is *shalom* (Judges 6:24). He it is who offers His people a covenant of *shalom*, that is, a covenant which will secure *shalom* for them (Numbers 25:12; Isaiah 54:10; Jeremiah 32:40; Ezekiel 34:25, 37:26; and Malachi 2:5). True *shalom* comes from God, for man [sic] finds his true wholeness and complete fulfilment only in God.[31]

Shalom is a person. Thus true health is not a particular state of mental or physical well-being (although it may include such things).

Rather health understood as *shalom* is a gift that God gives to His creation: a gift of God's self.

Jesus: Our *Shalom*

For the Hebrew prophets, the coming Messiah, the "Prince of Peace," would be the one who would return God's *shalom* to His people:

> The Messiah is the prince of *shalom* (Isa 9:6), he shall be the *shalom* (Micah 5:5), he shall speak *shalom* unto the heathen (Zech 9:10). . . . He will realise the plans of *shalom*, which the Lord has in mind for us, to give as a future and a hope.[32]

The Messiah will be the bringer and founder of the kingdom of peace. Which brings us back to Jesus. In the New Testament, the messianic mission of Jesus is closely linked to this understanding of God's Messiah as the bearer of *shalom*. It is Jesus, God's long awaited Messiah, who is the bearer and the sharer of Yahweh's *shalom*.[33] Thus, in the same way as in the Old Testament, "Yahweh is *Shalom*,"[34] so in the New Testament the apostle Paul informs his readers that Jesus is *Shalom*: "For *he himself* is our peace, who has made the two one and has destroyed the barrier, the dividing wall of hostility."[35]

Shalom is a person. Jesus *is shalom*. In John's Gospel, Jesus promises that he will give his *shalom*, his peace, to all those who would follow him:

> Peace I leave with you; my peace I give you. I do not give to you as the world gives. Do not let your hearts be troubled and do not be afraid.[36]

That being so, true health—*shalom*—is not something that can be understood outside of its true context in Jesus. That is the reason why my initial observations about the absence of Jesus from the religion and health research should be deeply concerning for Christians.

JESUS MATTERS

This theological perspective on the nature of health has important implications for the religion and health research agenda and the ways in which Christians should relate to it. It is clear theologically that bodies matter. If participation in religion brings about improvements in bodily well-being, then that can only be a good thing. God desires that His people flourish and care for their bodies and their minds. Indeed, as the apostle Paul points out, our bodies are the temple of the Holy Spirit, that is, the physical location of the Spirit of Jesus, the spirit of *shalom*.[37] If research can help us to see and understand the theological significance of the ways in which our beliefs and practices impact upon our well-being, it can effectively participate faithfully in God's redemptive *shalom*ic movement.

However, if such research serves only to bolster the genericization and medicalization of Christianity, then it misses the mark. To look only at one aspect of *shalom* without recognizing the implications for the whole is like examining the leg of an elephant without glancing upward to see that there may be more to it than immediately meets the eye. To reduce our explorations of religion and health to sets of behaviors, values, and psychological coping habits is interesting, but clearly theologically inadequate. Such explorations can only become theologically significant if and when they are recognized as taking place within a wider theological context—creation—within which the question, "What is health *for*?" takes on a quite particular shape and form. Health is Jesus and for Jesus.

CONCLUSION

My point then is not that we (the "we" here being the followers of Jesus) necessarily need to stop looking at the physiological or psychological effects of religion. We do, however, need to recontextualize such studies and place them in a wider theological framework within which their efficacy and faithfulness can be properly assessed. It makes a difference if I am a Christian, and that difference cannot and must not be reduced simply to behaviors and measurable observations of physiological changes.

Peter Berger calls for a deeper integration between theology and science. He states:

I would recommend that the scientific study of religion return to a perspective on the phenomenon "from within," that is, to viewing it in terms of the meanings intended by the religious consciousness.[38]

This chapter might be seen as a prolegomenon to such an enterprise. If we are to return to a perspective on the phenomenon "from within," it will be necessary to begin to develop what Abraham Maslow[39] has defined as an "expanded science"—a form of science that takes seriously issues of value, hope, meaning, and the unpredictable nature of lived experience and, I would add, the possibility that ultimate truth might not be as alien to the scientific exploration of religion and health as is often presumed. William James makes this point quite nicely:

[There are] many worlds of consciousness that exist . . . which have a meaning for our life. . . . The total expression of human experience . . . invincibly urges me beyond the narrow "scientific" bounds. Assuredly, the real world is of a different temperament—more intricately built than physical science allows.[40]

Such an approach will not exclude scientific methodology or the standard approaches of science, but it will help to put them in their proper context—*shalom*—and will work to develop, understand, and creatively utilize the types of theological and philosophical challenges that have been highlighted in this chapter.

What is required is rigorous, critical interdisciplinary dialogue carried out in a spirit of humility and hospitality: a mode of dialogue within which theology can help throw fresh light and understanding on the relationship between religion and health and within which the scientific research can help to clarify, challenge, and develop our understandings of what a practical theology of *shalom* might look like.

This chapter has urged Christians to bring Jesus into the conversation; to move from the general to the particular and to begin to redescribe the religion and health conversations in the light of *shalom*. This might be very difficult within a scientific context that prefers the general to the particular and that assumes that health is determined by what is measurable rather than the immeasurability of God's *shalom*. Nevertheless, with God all things are possible.[41]

NOTES

1. It is interesting to reflect on such a suggestion in the light of Koenig, McCulloch, and Larson's important collation of the evidence for the relationship between religion and health presented in their *Handbook of Religion and Health*. This book reviews over 1,600 studies and reviews on the effects of religion on health. The name of Jesus is mentioned only fourteen times, always in relation to research questionnaires, scales for measuring faith, or brief responses from research participants to the researcher's questions. This might not strike the reader as particularly odd until one reflects on precisely what it might mean to state that the Christian religion is good for your health without reference to the central figure without whom Christianity (and, as I will argue, health) makes no sense whatsoever. As we will see, this brief observation carries much theological importance. See Harold G. Koenig, Michael E. McCullough, and David B. Larson, *Handbook of Religion and Health (*New York: Oxford University Press, 2001).
2. Kenneth I. Pargament, "The Bitter and the Sweet: An Evaluation of the Costs and Benefits of Religiousness," *Psychological Inquiry* 13 (2002): 168–81.
3. Harold G. Koenig, ed., *Handbook of Religion and Mental Health* (San Diego: Academic Press, 1998), 112.
4. Attributed to Rev. William Ashley Sunday, quoted in *Greater Communications Effectiveness: Press, Radio, Television, Periodicals, Public Relations, and Advertising as Seen through Institutes and Special Occasions of the Henry W. Grady School of Journalism*, ed. John E. Drewry (Athens: University of Georgia Press, 1967).
5. Job 11:7, (NIV).
6. See 1 Corinthians 12:12–26 (NIV): "Just as a body, though one, has many parts, but all its many parts form one body, so it is with Christ. For we were all baptized by one Spirit so as to form one body—whether Jews or Gentiles, slave or free—and we were all given the one Spirit to drink. Even so the body is not made up of one part but of many. Now if the foot should say, 'Because I am not a hand, I do not belong to the body,' it would not for that reason stop being part of the body. And if the ear should say, 'Because I am not an eye, I do not belong to the body,' it would not for that reason stop being part of the body. If the whole body were an eye, where would the sense of hearing be? If the whole body were an ear, where would the sense of smell be? But in fact God has placed the parts in the body, every one of them, just as he wanted them to be. If they were all one part, where would the body be? As it is, there are many parts, but one body. The eye cannot say to the hand, 'I don't need you!' And the head cannot say to the feet, 'I don't need you!' On the contrary, those parts of the body that seem to be weaker are indispensable, and the parts that we think are less honorable we treat with special honor. And the parts that are unpresentable are treated with special modesty, while our presentable parts need no special treatment. But God has put the body together, giving greater honor to the parts that lacked it, so that there should be no division in the body, but that its parts should have equal concern for each other. If one part suffers, every part suffers with it; if one part is honored, every part rejoices with it."

7. One of the most methodologically sound research findings is the observation that participation in religious communities has health benefits. However, there is nothing special about this observation. Other human activities such as going to the theatre similarly facilitate health benefits. In other words, at the level of observing the health implications of religion, religion functions in exactly the same way that other forms of human activity do. See Koenraad Cuypers, Steinar Krokstad, Turid Lingaas Holmen, Margunn Skjei Knudtsen, Lars Olov Bygren, and Jostein Holmen, "Patterns of Receptive and Creative Cultural Activities and Their Association with Perceived Health, Anxiety, Depression and Satisfaction with Life among Adults: The HUNT Study, Norway," *Journal of Epidemiology and Community Health* (2011), online prepublication: 23 May 2011 doi:10.1136/jech.2010.113571.

8. See David Seedhouse, *Health: The Foundations for Achievement* (London: Wiley-Blackwell, 2001).

9. Michael E. McCullough, William T. Hoyt, David B. Larson, Harold G. Koenig, and Carl Thoresen, "Religious Involvement and Mortality: A Meta-Analytic Review," *Health Psychology* 19 (2000): 211–22.

10. Mario Timio, Giorgio Lippi, Sandro Venanzi, Simonetta Gentili, Guiseppe Quintaliani, Claudio Verdura, Claudio Monarca, Paolo Saronio, and Francesca Timio, "Blood Pressure Trend and Cardiovascular Events in Nuns in a Secluded Order: A 30-Year Follow-up Study," *Blood Pressure* 6 (1997): 81–87.

11. Yechiel Friedlander, Jeremy D. Kark, Nathan A. Kaufmann, and Yechezkiel Stein, "Coronary Heart Disease Risk Factors among Religious Groupings in a Jewish Population Sample in Jerusalem," *American Journal of Clinical Nutrition* 42 (1985): 511–21.

12. Andrea K. Shreve-Neiger and Barry A. Edelstein, "Religion and Anxiety: A Critical Review of the Literature," *Clinical Psychological Review* 24 (2004): 379–97.

13. Timothy B. Smith, Michael E. McCullough, and Justin Poll, "Religiousness and Depression: Evidence for a Main Effect and the Moderating Influence of Stressful Life Events," *Psychological Bulletin* 129 (2003): 614–36.

14. A. Autiero, "The Interpretation of Pain: The Point of View of Catholic Theology," *Acta Neurochirurgica Supplementum (Wien)* 38 (1987): 123–26.

15. Heidi W. F. M. de Gouw, Rudi G. J. Westendorp, Anton E. Kunst, Johan P. Mackenbach, and Jan P. Vandenbroucke, "Decreased Mortality among Contemplative Monks in The Netherlands," *American Journal of Epidemiology* 141 (1995): 771–75.

16. Thomas E. Oxman, Daniel H. Freeman Jr., and Eric D. Manheimer, "Lack of Social Participation or Religious Strength and Comfort as Risk Factors for Death after Cardiac Surgery in the Elderly," *Psychosomatic Medicine* 57 (1995): 5–15.

17. Elizabeth Knowles, *The Oxford Dictionary of Phrase and Fable* (London: Oxford University Press, 2006), 565.

18. In Michael Horace Barnes, ed., *Theology and the Social Sciences* (Maryknoll, NY: Orbis Books, 2000), 5.

19. Hebrews 11:1.

20. Brent D. Slife, Carolen Hope, and R. Scott Nebeker, "Examining the Relationship between Religious Spirituality and Psychological Science," *Journal of Humanistic Psychology* 39, no. 2 (1999): 51–85.

21. Herbert Benson, Jeffery A. Dusek, Jane B. Sherwood, Peter Lam, Charles F. Bethea, William Carpenter, Sidney Levitsky, Peter C. Hill, Donald W. Clem, Manoj K. Jain, David Drumel, Stephen L. Kopecky, Paul S. Mueller, Dean Marek, Sue Rollins, and Patricia L. Hibberd, "Study of the Therapeutic Effects of Intercessory Prayer (STEP) in Cardiac Bypass Patients: A Multicenter Randomized Trial of Uncertainty and Certainty of Receiving Intercessory Prayer," *American Heart Journal* 151 (2006): 934–42.

22. Dale A. Matthews, Sally M. Marlowe, and Francis S. MacNutt, "Effects of Intercessory Prayer on Patients with Rheumatoid Arthritis," *Southern Medical Journal* 93 (2000): 1177–86.

23. Luke 4:12 (NIV). See also Deuteronomy 6:16 (NIV): "Do not test the LORD your God as you did at Massah."

24. Peter L. Berger, *The Sacred Canopy: Elements of a Sociological Theory of Religion* (Garden City, NJ: Doubleday, 1967; New York: Anchor Press, 1990), 100.

25. Brent D. Slife, "Are the Methods of Psychology Compatible with Theism?" in *Why Psychology Needs Theology: A Radical-Reformation Perspective*, eds. Cameron Lee and Alvin Dueck (Grand Rapids, MI: Eerdmans, 2005), 168.

26. Peter L. Berger, "Some Second Thoughts on Substantive versus Functional Definitions of Religion," *Journal for the Scientific Study of Religion* 13 (1974): 125–33, quotation on 128.

27. See John Wilkinson, *Health & Healing* (Edinburgh, UK: Handsell Press, 1980), 5. For a further development of the concept of *shalom* in relation to mental health, see John Swinton, *From Bedlam to* Shalom*: Towards a Practical Theology of Human Nature, Interpersonal Relationships, and Mental Health Care* (New York: Peter Lang, 2000).

28. Wilkinson, *Health & Healing*, 5.

29. In John A. T. Robinson, *The Body, a Study in Pauline Theology* (Chicago: Alec R. Allenson, 1952), 14.

30. As the Westminster Shorter Catechism (Q.1) puts it: "What is the chief end of man [sic]? A. Man's chief end is to glorify God, and to enjoy him forever."

31. Wilkinson, *Health & Healing*, 5.

32. Johannes Christiaan Hoekendijk, *The Church Inside Out* (London: SCM Press, 1967), 19.

33. See John 14:27 (NIV): "Peace I leave with you; my peace I give you. I do not give to you as the world gives. Do not let your hearts be troubled and do not be afraid[95];" and John 16:33 (NIV): "I have told you these things, so that in me you may have peace. In this world you will have trouble. But take heart! I have overcome the world."

34. Judges 6:24.

35. Ephesians 2:14 (NIV); italics added. A juxtaposition of these two passages strongly suggests an affirmation of Jesus' divine nature and a consequent recognition of common purpose within the Trinity. This assertion that *shalom* is a common purpose of the Trinity becomes even more clear in the light of Galatians 5:22 (NIV) where one finds Paul asserting that the Spirit also is the bearer and sharer of *shalom*: "But the fruit of the Spirit is love, joy, peace, patience, kindness, goodness, faithfulness."

36. John 14:27 (NIV).

37. 1 Corinthians 6:19 (NIV): "Do you not know that your body is a temple of the Holy Spirit, who is in you, whom you have received from God? You are not your own."

38. Berger, "Some Second Thoughts on Substantive versus Functional Definitions of Religion," 129.

39. Abraham Maslow, *The Farther Reaches of Human Nature* (New York: Penguin Books, 1985).

40. William James, *The Varieties of Religious Experience: A Study in Human Nature* [1902] (New York: Mentor, 1958), 391.

41. Matthew 19:26 (NIV): "Jesus looked at them and said, 'With man this is impossible, but with God all things are possible.'"

STANLEY HAUERWAS

10. *SUFFERING PRESENCE*

Twenty-Five Years Later

LOOKING BACK

The title of this essay intentionally mimics an essay I wrote some time ago entitled "The Narrative Turn: Thirty Years Later."[1] In the essay on narrative I revisited the general theme so determinative for how I think, that is, that knowledge of God and knowledge of the self is best displayed through narratives. I used the opportunity to assess the "turn to narrative" in order to distance myself from what I thought were some of the doubtful apologetic and popular uses of "story theology." In particular, I worried that the emphasis on story could reproduce habits associated with foundational theological projects that too often result in anthropological reductive accounts of theological claims. I was not then, nor am I now, suggesting that I think the attention to narrative for displaying the grammar of theological work to be a mistake, but rather I meant only to remind myself and those influenced by what I had said about narrative that theological appeals to narrative are not an end in itself.

Suffering Presence: Theological Reflections on Medicine, the Mentally Handicapped, and the Church was published in 1986. I am going to use this opportunity to write about the relation of theology and medicine to look again at what I was trying to do in that book. I wish I could say that this retrospective look back to the publication of that book was meant to serve the same purpose as my essay about narrative theology, that is, to counter some of the enthusiasm engendered by the publication of that book twenty-five years ago.[2] But *Suffering Presence* is a book that, as far as I can judge, fell stillborn from the press.[3] That it did so is not surprising. After all, I was trying to challenge some of the dominant paradigms associated with the development of medical ethics. From my perspective the development of medical ethics was but a legitimating discourse to underwrite, as Joel Shuman would later argue in a more sustained way, the transformation of medicine into an "industry that is in the business of selling an especially desirable product, namely health."[4]

I risk being self-indulgent by directing attention to my past work, but by doing so I hope to suggest that there is a connection between "the narrative turn" and how the relation of theology and medicine should be understood. By making explicit some of the intuitions that informed what I was trying to do in *Suffering Presence*, I hope I can say better now what I had tried to say then about how the body that is the subject of illness and death is a storied body. That it is so, moreover, means that any attempt to care for the body that fails to so recognize the storied character of our bodies cannot help but distort the gesture of presence called medicine.

By developing this understanding of the body, I hope it may help us say better what role a person's faith makes for responding to illness and the care and healing of the ill, but that is not my primary interest. I am sure the religious convictions patients and physicians bring to their encounters can and sometimes do make a difference for the character of those interactions. I have no doubt that prayer can and does make a difference when we are ill. I worry, however, that to emphasize the difference that prayer makes may lead to our forgetting that prayer has been given to us, not to make a difference even when we are sick, but in order that we might acknowledge the difference God has made by choosing to be our God. My subject, therefore, is not the difference "religion" can make for the recovery from illness. Rather I understand my task to be a normative one, that is, I want to try to say how Christians should care for one another through the office of medicine.

My argument assumes, using the title of Wendell Berry's wonderful chapter "Health Is Membership" in *Another Turn of the Crank*, that health is just that, namely, membership in a community.[5] Berry's insight about health as membership may seem, like much he has to say, a commonplace, but I hope to show it is a commonplace that is a deep challenge to the practice of contemporary medicine. For medicine as a practice in advanced societies like the United States cannot acknowledge that it reflects the material conditions of any particular community.

The irony, of course, is that medicine does reflect the material conditions of a particular community, but it is a community dominated by economic and political ideologies that claim to be first and foremost about securing the freedom of the individual. As a consequence, anonymity becomes a way of life and as a result many of our interactions with one another cannot help but be manipulative.[6] In a world in which it is assumed we share no goods in common, medicine cannot help but seem to be but another impersonal institution that delivers services to consumers. Ironically, a medicine so determined cannot acknowledge that the body, which allegedly is the subject of the medical arts, is a storied body. For a storied body is not the body of "anyone," but the body determined by a particular history of a particular community.

If the body is appropriately understood as a storied body, Berry argues that no hard-and-fast distinction can be drawn between the physical and the spiritual. That we currently make that distinction, according to Berry, only reflects how an understanding of the body as a machine has come to dominate our lives and, in particular, medical care. As a result Berry describes the contemporary hospital as a place where the world of love meets the world of efficiency, that is, the world of specialization, machinery, and abstract procedures, in a manner that those worlds are relegated to separate spheres.[7] At best love can be expressed in such a context primarily as the attempt to get the "best medical care available," but the "best medical care available" is not determined by a community of love.

These are complex matters that easily invite misunderstanding. *Suffering Presence* was written before I had read Berry, but I think it is quite compatible with Berry's understanding of health as membership. For example, in *Suffering Presence* I argued that medicine is an office of a community in which some are set aside to be present to the sick even when they cannot cure the person who is sick. I should like to think that understanding of the role of medicine to be quite similar to the way Berry depicts the mutual responsibilities of the physician and patient.

I have been criticized for allegedly assuming a far too idealized account of medicine. I understand the worry because such a view of medicine seems to have little relation to the reality of the medical care currently practiced. I was not, however, trying to suggest that we must find a way to recover the medicine practiced by the "small town doctor." The medicine we have is the medicine we have. Modern medicine can be quite brutal, but so could the medicine of the past. It is my judgment, however, that the actual practice of medicine, even a medicine determined by the demands of efficiency, is often more "humane" than it is given credit.

That Berry understands health to be a concept that draws on a more determinative sense of community, however, is the reason his reflections on illness are formed by stories. Berry remains far too close to the ground to forget that no matter what we may say about who we "really are," who we "really are" is most determinatively indicated by our bodies in relation to other bodies. For Berry, when our bodies are abstracted from the communities that constitute the trust and love that give life, we have an exemplification of an abstract understanding of the body that can only be destructive.[8]

A body so determined may invite a concern about "spirituality" when that body needs to be healed. But a spirituality (and religion) divorced from the actual practices that shape the body threatens to be far too generic to do any serious work if serious work is understood to be the work of Christian theology.[9] "Health" may even be a more ambiguous term than spirituality. When "health" is thought to name "total well-being," as it often is in modernity, and medicine becomes the agent of health, this threatens to make medicine the institution of a secular salvation.[10] I suspect that is why for many today medicine has become an alternative church.

This assessment formed the background for the case I tried to develop in *Suffering Presence* where I called for a practice of medicine that subordinated medical care to the determinative ends of a community. Of course, the community with which I was principally concerned is called "church." The emphasis on the body as the proper subject of medical care in *Suffering Presence* was an attempt to suggest why a church must exist if the care we provide to one another through the office of medicine is to be kept within appropriate limits. While I think that emphasis is needed, in my attempt to highlight the hubris of modern medicine I failed to say enough about the body that is the proper subject of medicine.

That hubris—that is, the presumption that through medicine we can get out of life alive—is not the fault of physicians. Rather that expectation, admittedly an expectation that physicians and researchers have encouraged and from which they have benefited, is carried by patients who are anything but patient.[11] Ironically, the spiritualization of the body, a denial of the finite character that is our body, a denial often legitimated by Christian "beliefs," means that the body patients ask physicians to care for is not the body shaped by the body of Christ.[12]

I wrote *Suffering Presence*, therefore, in an effort to remind us that medical ethics is not a disciplined mode of reflection about how physicians should act toward patients. For I take it that medicine names not only what physicians do but it is a determinative interaction between doctor and patient. The focus on patients for determining how we should think about the ends of medicine, therefore, was at the heart of the fundamental perspective I tried to develop in *Suffering Presence*. We will not get a more modest medicine in service to the body until we recognize that as patients for good or ill we get the medicine we deserve. Let me try to explain this last remark by suggesting some of the problems that currently seem to bedevil communication between patients and physicians in our day.

BARRIERS TO COMMUNICATION BETWEEN DOCTORS AND PATIENTS

It is often forgotten that physicians are human beings. Because physicians are human beings, they—like their patients—would like to be liked. Translated into the grammar of medicine, this desire to be liked means physicians would like to help those who are sick and seek their help. This desire becomes problematic when the patient has been formed to expect "cures" that the physician cannot honestly provide. The sick seek out physicians because they rightly think a physician knows what needs to be known to help them and can do what needs to be done to make what is threatening them less threatening. The problem is quite simply that, given the reality physicians confront on a daily basis, they know what their patients know but do not want to acknowledge, that is, when it is all said and done we are all going to die. Patients, however, often do not or cannot acknowledge that reality and as a result subject physicians to expectations that cannot be met.

The tension between what the patient expects and what the physician can do is complicated by the recognition that at least one aspect of the therapy a physician represents is the trust the patient has in the physician. If the physician seems to be in doubt about what is wrong with the patient, even more what might be an appropriate intervention, patients can feel betrayed, making it even more difficult for the physician to speak truthfully to their patients. This is complicated by the vast differences that education, class, gender, and race present for communication between physician and patient. Essays like the ones in this book are written by highly educated people who assume that most patients a physician deals with are like them, that is, highly educated. But physicians do not care only for the highly educated. They also care for people who do not know what blood pressure names.

Yet the physician, at least in theory, is obligated to care for a patient no matter what their educational level or race may be. Medicine, for all of its problems, remains an extraordinary morally formed practice. That is why in *Suffering Presence* I suggested that the very idea that physicians needed to be taught "ethics" to sustain their work only leads to a distortion of the ethics that is constitutive of the physicians' work. Fundamental to that ethic is the presumption that a physician is to care for the patient before them in a manner that makes all other considerations irrelevant. That commitment I take to be at the heart of the trust that should characterize the relation between a physician and their patient. The patient must have confidence that the care they are receiving will not be subject to considerations of what they can pay, what another patient may need, or whether the physician does or does not like them. So the physician is caught. They must care for patients in a manner commensurate with their training and skills, but the patient may well not appreciate the limits of what the physician can do.

The account of medicine I provided in *Suffering Presence* was meant to be a response to this unhappy state of affairs by developing an account of authority that legitimates the physician's care of another human being even when that care cannot "cure." I developed that suggestion by calling attention to the "authority of the body." I even suggested that by focusing on the body I was exploring a kind of natural law reasoning shaped by our bodily character. For at least one of the aspects we share as human beings is that we are bodies. Moreover, that we are bodies makes possible the interactions necessary to discover the goods we have in common. To be sure, those goods are mediated by traditions that are diverse and often in conflict, but to the extent we share in having bodies means we have some basis for mutual recognition.

Accordingly, I argued that "medicine is the name for a tradition of wisdom concerning good care of the body. As such it is not a 'means' to health, but rather is part of the activity of health—an activity that involves as much participation of the patient as the physician."[13] The body sets a norm for medicine because the body is classically understood as the artist of its own healing. The task of those in medicine is to aid us in living through our bodies because it is a mistake—a mistake, I fear, that may ironically be characteristic of the celebration of the body in modernity—to try to live beyond our bodies.

In *Suffering Presence* I argued that in contrast to such an understanding of the body, medicine is, therefore, best understood as an ongoing tradition of wisdom and practices through which physicians acquire the responsibility to remember, learn, and pass on the skills of learning to live with a body that is destined to death.[14] To sustain medicine so understood would require a community that was capable of resisting the seduction of what I can only characterize as the Gnosticism of modernity.

The focus on the body, a body that is not simply a physical body but a lived body, was my attempt to show how physician and patient alike share a common good that could at once limit as well as legitimate physician intervention. By calling attention to how the body can act as an "authority," I sought a way to help physician and patient to discover a common language, making communication possible. In particular, I commended Eric Cassell's account of the physician's task to be first and foremost to educate their patients to acknowledge their bodies.[15]

BODY MATTERS

I continue to think I was on the right track by directing attention to the body as the locus for the kind of discourse necessary to legitimate the work of medicine. But I confess I was trying to have my cake and eat it too. I was trying to show how the body can provide a necessary limit to our desires for escaping finitude while also suggesting the difference Christian formation makes for the care we provide for one another through the office of medicine. Because I believe that to be a Christian is the fullest expression of what it means to be a human being, I do not think these two emphases necessarily to be in tension. But given the imperative of the Baconian project, we cannot assume the body Christians believe is a gift from God is the same body that shapes modern medicine.[16]

Jeffrey P. Bishop, for example, argues in his book, *The Anticipatory*

Corpse: Medicine, Power, and the Care of the Dying, that the body that determines the care provided by modern medicine is the corpse.[17] That a medical students' encounter with their first patient is an encounter with a corpse Bishop takes to be a sign of how the body is generally understood in modern medicine. According to Bishop, at least since Bacon, it has been assumed that the body, like the world itself, is essentially without purpose other than our ability to impose on it our arbitrary desires. The body is therefore understood as a malleable object subject only to instrumental causation.

Given this mechanistic understanding of life, Bishop argues that the care, particularly of the dying, provided by modern medicine is built on a metaphysics of efficient causation made possible by the epistemological assumption that true knowledge of the body is knowledge of the dead body. In contrast, knowledge of a lived body, a body that to be sure is transitory, makes a science of medicine difficult because a lived body is an unpredictable body.

That is why Bishop suggests that the body presupposed by research medicine is the dead body because a dead body makes possible predicable knowledge. Bishop concludes, "The dead body is the measure of medicine, creating the sense that life is primarily matter ordered to efficiently move within space, both within the space of the body itself but also within space of the body politic."[18]

I am sure many may think Bishop has overstated his argument. Surely the body that is at the center of medical care is the lived body. After all, the subject of medical art is not the body but a bodily patient. The body that the patient presents to the physician, moreover, is a storied body that physicians soon learn they must listen to if they are to care for the patient. Yet it is surely the case that there is a tension between the science of the body presumed by research medicine and the everyday practice of medicine. Jerome Groopman illustrates that tension by calling attention to Dr. Myron Falchuk's observation that patients come to him as a specialist who is able to perform a procedure using a specialized technology. The technology is vital for caring for the patient, but Falchuk observes, "I believe that this technology also has taken us away from the patient's story. And once you remove yourself from the patient's story, you no longer are truly a doctor."[19]

Increasing medical specialization may be an indication that the body that shapes medical care is, as Bishop maintains, a dead body. For a lived body means there is no way to avoid judgments about patients that may prove to be mistaken.[20] The uncertainty associated with primary care may well be one of the reasons that many physicians try to avoid that "specialty." But specialization serves only to give those in the diverse specializations of medicine a false sense of certainty because specialization can result in a failure to "see" the patient.[21] To be able to see the patient, one has to listen to the patient.

As specializations increasingly correspond to technological developments, specializations also occasion both critical and constructive reflections on the physician-patient relationship as it is affected by technology. Many fear that technology contributes to a further distancing between doctor and patient. But Atul Gawande observes that compassion and technology are not incompatible and may even be mutually reinforcing. The machine may make mistakes less likely and, he notes, nothing is more disruptive of the relation between a patient and a doctor than a mistake.

Of course, as Gawande acknowledges, machines can and do make mistakes, but as "systems" take on the more technical work of medicine, technologies can free physicians to embrace dimensions of care that mattered prior to the development of technology, such as talking to their patients. To talk to patients is necessary because, as he puts it, "medical care is about our life and death, and we have always needed doctors to help us understand what is happening and why, and what is possible and what is not. In the increasingly tangled web of experts and expert systems, a doctor has an even greater obligation to serve as a knowledgeable guide and confident. Maybe machines can decide, but we still need doctors to heal."[22]

Gawande is right: we do need doctors to heal. But if Bishop is also right, then the "healing" that physicians provide may be determined by an understanding of the body that is in tension with the lived body of the patient. Therefore, I think it important to say explicitly what I only hinted at in *Suffering Presence*. If the Christian body is first and foremost a body meant to glorify God, then Christians must begin to contemplate that the kind of medicine that should characterize the Christian body may be quite different from that which does not share the practices of the church. In short, I think that Christians may well find that they will need to develop a medicine that reflects the Christian difference. For the body the church presents to be cared for is not the isolated body of strangers but the baptized body of the people of God. That body, the baptized body, is shaped by practices carried by the story of God in which illness, suffering, and death are not regarded as the ultimate enemy. They cannot be regarded as the ultimate enemy because Christians believe that even our suffering can be a gift that makes more intimate our relation with God and one another.[23]

THE CHRISTIAN BODY

I indicated above that the body that presents itself to a physician is a lived body. A "lived" body is a storied body. This is why my earlier essay on narrative is relevant to the case I tried to make in *Suffering Presence*. Our bodies demand habituation through which we acquire, as Aristotle argued, "a second nature."[24] If brought up rightly, that "nature" makes possible the acquisition of the habits we call the virtues. How the virtues and their interrelation are understood reflect the stories that shape the fundamental practices of the communities in which we live. For Christians, health itself is a virtue that makes possible our presence to one another in health, sickness, and suffering. Health, like all the virtues, is a reflection of the love of God.[25]

Indeed, a Christian view of health does not deny that some among us are sick and will need care. Rather, a Christian view of health requires that the community recognize illness so that the one who is sick may be restored to health, but more importantly so that the one who is sick remains part of the community even if their health is not restored. This means that the Christian view of health forms patients who want to be cured but are not seeking that cure at all costs. In other words, the Christian view of health entails the understanding that the Christian difference means being at peace with human finitude—and even seeing human finitude as a gift.

Conversely, Christian health also means it may be appropriate for Christians to hold one another accountable when choices are being made that negatively affect one's health such that they are inhibited from participating fully in service to God and world. From this perspective, Christian health doesn't mean the absence of illness but the reliance on Christ and his community, the church, even while facing the realities of illness and death. It is this faithfulness to Christ that marks the difference of Christian suffering and it is but a response to Christ's faithfulness to us—even in the midst of his own suffering. Like Christ, Christians must learn how to suffer without losing hope. We must learn to pray for our physicians, not only that they might have the knowledge to help us, but that they might have the courage to tell us when they cannot. Even more, we must learn to forgive them when they lack the courage. And, finally, we must learn to sit with one another in the valley of the shadow of death.

By suggesting that we need to attend to the Christian difference I am not trying to argue that difference is as an end in itself. Rather I'm suggesting that the Christian difference should determine how Christians understand the role and office of medicine. As I argued in *Suffering Presence*, for a community to set aside some to be with the sick is an extraordinary gesture that draws on a profound sense of the significance of presence to one another as a defining mark of the church. That presence, moreover, is made possible through a shared language, and language of the body, that makes communication between the doctor and their patient possible.

I do not mean to suggest that the formation of physicians by the church would restrict them to only caring for Christians. But if a Christian doctor believes they must speak truthfully to their patient, non-Christians might begin to worry whether they want a doctor who is a Christian. This is not simply because a physician who is a Christian will not perform an abortion or entertain the possibility of euthanasia.

Those kinds of concerns certainly matter, but I am suggesting more than this. If "health is membership," the very isolation that the doctor-patient relation too often enacts has to be reconsidered.

Formed by the presumptions of modern medicine, I fear that the way Christians pray indicates there is too often very little difference between how Christians approach illness than non-Christians. The god to whom we pray when we are ill I fear is too often a "god of the gaps," that is, the god to whom we pray is a deistic god who exists, it seems, to be an insurance policy to protect us from the unknown. But that god cannot be the One who came in the flesh so that we not despise our flesh that beacons our deaths.

The God we worship as Christian taught us to pray, "Thy will be done." We even believe that the Holy Spirit prays on our behalf when, in the face of suffering, we are unable to pray for ourselves. I am suggesting that the Christian difference means our prayers are not determined by the valley of the shadow of death, but rather they are determined by the presence of the One that walks with us. The story that determines the Christian body is the story of Emmanuel, God with us. This is the story we were baptized into, which means we have already died. Therefore, the hope we share is ultimately not a hope to get through life unscathed—but a hope to remain faithful until the end. It is the hope of the resurrection.

A medicine understood as an office of that community called church means the "and" between theology and medicine cannot represent two quite distinct activities that must now be related. Rather the "and" indicates the task of the church to be the kind of community that can sustain the care of the bodies we share through the office of medicine.

Illness usually comes as an unexpected guest, threatening to disorder our routines and make our lives incoherent. The stories that constitute our lives are meant to give us a sense of control and to assure us we know where we are and in what time we live. Yet the stories that we may actually be living may not be the ones we think we are living, but our illusions are dear to us. Illness often destroys our illusions as well as our confidence that we are in control. To be a Christian is to undergo the training necessary to know how to live out of control. Accordingly, to suffer those that suffer bonds those who are currently not sick to those that are sick through a common story, making possible the acknowledgment that even the suffering of those we love cannot separate us from the love of God.

A medical care shaped by such a people does not need to promise "cure" to have authority or legitimacy. The care of one another in the name of medicine does not even need to promise "restoration." Rather what such a medicine promises, the trust it instills, is to reflect through its care of the sick, the story into which we were baptized. Such a community must be capable of supporting physicians who can tell us that they have no idea what may be wrong with us, but they will continue to care for us. Such a community must be capable of sustaining physicians who are able to acknowledge that practicing the best medicine they know will sometimes entail making a mistake. Such a community is able to sustain a practice of medicine so conceived because patient and physician alike have been made participants in a common story.

For many, what I am calling for will seem unrealistic given the character of the contemporary church, as well as the power of modern medicine. However I think the way I am trying to help us think about our care of one another through the office of medicine as Christians can be in continuity with the everyday reality of church life. For the everyday reality of church life is to participate in the worship of God and in the process to discover the storied character of our lives. We have been given what we need, but we can lose what we have been given because we have been captured by other narratives that tempt us to describe our lives in terms foreign to the Gospel.

In his memoir, *The Pastor*, Eugene H. Peterson provides an account of the formation of a congregation that suggests what I am trying to imagine can be possible.[26] Peterson, who had not intended to be a "pastor," found himself in the process of starting a new church. He soon discovered he had no idea who would show up from one Sunday to another Sunday. Not all who came stayed, but as the church grew, he observes, something like a story began to develop that shaped the self-understanding of those that shared the worship of God. Reflecting on this development, Peterson observes that when we get caught up in a story, if it is a truthful story, we do not know how it might end and/or who else will become part of the story.[27] The storied character of a congregation and the storied character of our lives are inextricably interrelated as they involve discoveries we had not anticipated—discoveries that occur through our living together.

Peterson is candid that the church that was coming into being was not an ideal church, but a church made up of human beings. They were people who became ill and died. And those illnesses and deaths became part of the story that made Christ Our King the body of Christ. Peterson observes that this reality was made possible because the stories that constitute Christ Our King church provide a language in which everyone is organically related through the discoveries of "patterns and meanings—beauty and truth and goodness: Father, Son, and Holy Spirit. In the seemingly random and disconnected pieces of experience and dream, tasks and songs, promises and betrayals that make up daily life, words and sentences detect and fashion stories in places of hospitality."[28]

I should like to think the church Peterson describes is one I was trying to imagine twenty-five years ago in *Suffering Presence*. Physicians and patients, whether they are Christian or not, find that we are increasingly trapped in a medical system that is not sustainable and may well be self-destructing. So we have little to lose if Christians begin to try to imagine what it might mean to form our care of one another through a medicine that respects the body that is storied by Christ.

NOTES

1. Stanley Hauerwas, *Performing the Faith: Bonhoeffer and the Practice of Nonviolence* (Grand Rapids: Brazos Press, 2004), 135–50.
2. Stanley Hauerwas, *Suffering Presence: Theological Reflections on Medicine, the Mentally Handicapped, and the Church* (Notre Dame, IN: University of Notre Dame Press, 1986).

3. I am, however, particularly grateful to Gerald P. McKenny for his insightful account and critique of my work in his book *To Relieve the Human Condition: Bioethics, Technology, and the Body* (Albany: State University of New York, 1997), 147–83.

4. Joel James Shuman, *The Body of Compassion: Ethics, Medicine, and the Church* (Boulder, CO: Westview Press, 1999), 10.

5. Wendell Berry, *Another Turn of the Crank* (Washington, DC: Counterpoint, 1995), 86–109.

6. Alasdair MacIntyre's account of the relationship of bureaucracy and the manipulative character of human relationship in a liberal culture remains unsurpassed but unfortunately not sufficiently acknowledged for the significance of his insights. See his *After Virtue: A Study in Moral Theology*, 3rd ed. (Notre Dame, IN: University of Notre Dame Press, 2007), 23–35.

7. Berry, *Another Turn of the Crank*, 102.

8. For a wonderful overview of Berry's work, see Fritz Oehlschlaeger, *The Achievement of Wendell Berry: The Hard History of Love* (Lexington: University of Kentucky Press, 2011).

9. For my worries about "religion," see the chapter, "The End of 'Religious Pluralism': A Tribute to David Burrell," in my *The State of the University: Academic Knowledges and the Knowledge of God* (Oxford, UK: Blackwell, 2007), 58–75. More significant is William Cavanaugh's argument in *The Myth of Religious Violence: Secular Ideology and the Roots of Modern Conflict* (Oxford, UK: Oxford University Press, 2009) to the effect that the very creation of the category of religion went hand in hand with the attempt to legitimate the modern nation-state as the necessary alternative to the alleged wars of religion.

10. In 1948, the newly founded World Health Organization defined health as "a state of complete physical, mental, and social well-being and not merely the absence of disease or infirmity." The list has been expanded to include emotional, intellectual, physical, environmental, social, occupational, and spiritual aspects of health. I am indebted to Melanie Dobson Hughes for calling my attention to the WHO account of health.

11. See my "Practicing Patience: How Christians Should Be Sick," in my and Charles R. Pinches' *Christians Among the Virtues: Theological Conversations with Ancient and Modern Ethics* (Notre Dame, IN: University of Notre Dame Press, 1997), 166–78.

12. I am indebted to Keith Meador for this point.

13. Hauerwas, *Suffering Presence*, 47.

14. Ibid., 48.

15. Ibid., 49. Eric Cassell's book is *The Healers Art: A New Approach to the Doctor-Patient Relationship* (Philadelphia: Lippincott, 1976).

16. For an account of the Baconian project, see McKenny, *To Relieve the Human Condition*, 25–38.

17. Jeffrey P. Bishop, *The Anticipatory Corpse: Medicine, Power, and the Care of the Dying* (Notre Dame, IN: University of Notre Dame Press, 2011).

18. Ibid., 21–22.

19. Quoted in Jerome Groopman, *How Doctors Think* (Boston: Houghton Mifflin, 2007), 16–17.

20. Atul Gawande observes: "We look for medicine to be an orderly field of knowledge and procedure. But it is not. It is an imperfect science, an enterprise of constantly changing knowledge, uncertain information, fallible individuals, and at the same time lives on the line. There is science in what we do, yes, but also habit, intuition, and sometimes plain old guessing. The gap between what we know and what we aim for persists. And this gap complicates everything we do." In *Complications: A Surgeon's Notes on an Imperfect Science* (New York: Picador, 2002), 7.

21. Groopman, *How Doctors Think*, 152–55.

22. Gawande, *Complications*, 45–46.

23. For a defense of this understanding of suffering, see Eleonore Stump, *Wandering in Darkness: Narrative and the Problem of Suffering* (New York: Oxford University Press, 2010).

24. Aristotle, *Nicomachean Ethics* [c. 350 BCE], 2nd ed., trans. Terence Irwin (Indianapolis: Hackett, 1999), 1103a15–35.

25. Aquinas understands health to be a virtue, but he provides an extremely sensitive account, noting that the measure of health is not the same in all or even in one individual. Accordingly, a person may be sick but still embody the virtue of health. Health is a habit and like all habits health can be greater or less; see *The Summa Theologica of St. Thomas Aquinas* [c. 1274], trans. Fathers of the English Dominican Province (Westminster, MD: Christian Classics, 1948), I-II, 52, 1.

26. Eugene H. Peterson, *The Pastor: A Memoir* (New York: HarperCollins, 2011), 118–19.

27. Ibid., 118.

28. Ibid., 309.

KEITH G. MEADOR

EPILOGUE. THEOLOGY AND HEALTH

Challenges and Possibilities

CHALLENGES

Many of the authors in this book have noted the proliferation of research in religion and health research in the last two decades. In response to the invitation extended to our authors as framed by my coeditor in the prologue, authors from both the Jewish and Christian communities have richly enhanced the conversation of religion and health with their thoughtful, pastorally formed responses and incisive theological critiques. While not intending to summarize nor lend commentary on all of the essays that so substantially stand on their own, I do want to note the contributions made by some of the authors in this book, bearing witness to the concerns noted and shared by many of us interested in religion and health. These concerns can perhaps most constructively be expressed as the hope and anticipation that the current movement in religion and health, with all of its diversity and intensity, will not just be an interesting sociological phenomenon of the late twentieth and early twenty-first centuries, but rather will offer a prophetic voice that challenges and transforms our cultural understandings of health and the practice of medicine in care of the suffering among us for many years to come due to its intellectual rigor and theological integrity. We hope this book makes a distinctive contribution in supporting both, but particularly the latter, within the Jewish and Christian traditions.

Rabbi Address thoughtfully orients us when stating, "At the root of all of these exhortations, edicts, and interpretations is the fundamental understanding that we are to take care of our health and bodies and life so as to be able to be in relationship with God."[1] One of the great theological distortions of the religion and health movement has been its proclivity to reverse this statement explicitly or by inference to indicate that we are to be in "relationship with God," or spiritual by some measure, so as to gain health and well-being, as if this were the primary purpose of love and obedience to God. While there is, and should be, much discussion as to the implications of such claims within both the academic and popular culture, the centrality of its place in the religion and health conversation is inevitable in our current outcomes-based interpretation of the relationship of religion and health whereby "outcomes" are determined by the prevailing empirically driven consumerist-based biomedical enterprise.

Complementary to Rabbi Address' perspective but coming from the Christian tradition, John Swinton notes in his chapter the biblical use of the word *shalom* to embody much of what the current religion and health movement would ascribe to "health":

> However, such health is important only as it contributes to the ongoing implementation of God's *shalom*. The fact that religion is good for your medical health only has significance if one recognizes what such health is *for*: the glory of God. Bodies matter, but only as they orient people toward the true source of health: Jesus.[2]

Multiple authors in this book have examined various dimensions of this issue and its implications. While legitimate arguments can be made defending against the concerns others and I have voiced through the years regarding instrumentalizing religion and spirituality in service to health,[3] persistently subtle, if not overt, tendencies toward distortions of both health and religion inherent to the religion and health movement of the last two decades are manifested within this instrumentalization. The religion and health research agenda—of which many of us have been a part—has unquestionably contributed to this process, but the broadly embraced cultural synergies of the presumptions embedded within the consumerist impulses of American Protestantism as a whole and the contemporary "prosperity gospel" in particular facilitates the appropriation of this instrumental use of religion and spirituality as part of the marketing of religion and spirituality as a means to health and well-being as construed by contemporary culture. While most of us within major faith traditions have some sense of religion and spirituality positively contributing to the "*shalom*" of participants within these communities of practice consistent with the empirical findings to date, gaining a better understanding of the processes and patterns of influence by which this contribution is made begs for a more theologically astute and informed methodology.

Substantive and discernibly credible claims regarding the potential "mechanisms" by which religion and health are related demand a more robust and methodologically sophisticated inclusion of the relevant particularities embedded within specific traditions of belief and practice. While the lure of some form of generalizable spirituality for research design purposes is seductive and understandably appealing when designing research tools and instruments, the implications of such efforts are theologically suspect and leave theologically discerning critics questioning the validity of such empirically derived claims regarding the relationship between religion and health. Notably, the domestication of God embodied within this appropriation of generic spirituality common to the religion and health research enterprise is not the exclusive domain of the empirical research agenda. It has been promulgated, frequently with enthusiasm while somewhat unknowingly, by religious and spiritual participants and enthusiasts themselves, thus perpetuating the presumption by researchers that it is an acceptable practice. Intriguingly, an astute observer of human nature, albeit not one known for concerns regarding loss of religiosity, Sigmund Freud, noted in his *The Future of an Illusion*:

Where questions of religion are concerned, people are guilty of every possible sort of dishonesty and intellectual misdemeanor. . . . They give the name of "God" to some vague abstraction which they have created for themselves; having done so they can pose before all the world as deists, as believers in God, and they can even boast that they have recognized a higher, purer concept of God, notwithstanding that their God is now nothing more than an insubstantial shadow and no longer the mighty personality of religious doctrines.[4]

Even Freud with his skepticism regarding religious belief in general could discern and critique the domestication and reduction of God to the "insubstantial shadow" frequently reflected in the "higher powers" to which generic spirituality frequently finds itself appealing in seeking a relationship to health. Through the lens of the particular traditions of Judaism and Christianity our authors have consistently, yet with diversity of approaches, sought to elucidate the importance of theological particularity in intellectual engagement and pastoral practice. This commitment is understood to be manifested within communities of faith and practice in order to avoid the theological distortion of employing a domesticated God in an instrumentalized use of spirituality and religion in service to individualistic consumerist impulses of personal spirituality.

Parallel and interwoven with this theological distortion, through the domestication of God leading to a misguided use of instrumentalism and generic spirituality in the religion and health movement, we see a distorted understanding of "health" to which I alluded earlier when commenting on Swinton's challenges to the movement. This issue merits further focused consideration. The religion and health literature struggles to find the best "health" outcome to use in relation to religion and spirituality and then is frequently challenged in its efforts to adequately measure the outcome chosen. In seeking to best understand the relationship of religion and health, the outcomes may be less concrete than such standard measures as mortality or discrete assessments of typical medical illnesses. The cross-sectional epidemiologic literature examining such outcomes as mortality in relation to religion is informative but limited in its possibilities for nuanced understandings of the relationship.

I would join our theological colleagues who challenge us to develop a much richer and textured understanding of health, incorporating such language and conceptual frameworks as human flourishing with an understanding that one might humanly flourish even while dying and facing one's inevitable mortality. How can we gain a better understanding of religion and health in the context of the inevitable decline and mortality inherent to "the human condition"?[5] Stanley Hauerwas frames this perspective well in his chapter from within the Christian tradition, saying:

> Our bodies demand habituation through which we acquire, as Aristotle argued, "a second nature." If brought up rightly, that "nature" makes possible the acquisition of the habits we call the virtues. . . . Health, like all the virtues, is a reflection of the love of God.
>
> Indeed, a Christian view of health does not deny that some among us are sick and will need care. Rather, a Christian view of health requires that the community recognize illness so that the one who is sick may be restored to health, but more importantly so that the one who is sick remains part of the community even if their health is not restored. This means that the Christian view of health forms patients who want to be cured but are not seeking that cure at all costs. In other words, the Christian view of health entails the understanding that the Christian difference means being at peace with human finitude—and even seeing human finitude as a gift.[6]

Such an understanding of health challenges simplistic outcome measures that would attempt to use standard epidemiologic survey methods to ascertain health in relation to religion and spirituality. Measuring "peace with human finitude" is challenging and may be unattainable, but the theological challenge to acknowledge such refinements in our understanding of health are crucial. Warren Kinghorn rightly challenges us in his chapter to engage the language of "human flourishing," developing his use of this notion within his work with Aquinas and stating that "a Thomistically informed 'religion and health' movement would understand itself, most broadly, as a science of human flourishing. Such a movement would want to know what sorts of bodily and psychological configurations reflect and/or contribute to flourishing, and what sorts of these configurations detract from it."[7]

While many in the academic religion and health community have struggled with the measurement challenges regarding religiosity or spirituality through the years, the parallel challenge of adequately discerning and measuring the appropriate "health" outcome for religion and health research has not been as consistently considered. In order to optimally engage this issue we must give attention to the particular goods valued by divergent traditions and communities as they discern "flourishing" within their respective worldviews. The degree to which religion and spirituality contribute to such flourishing is contingent upon the measure of health ultimately used and determined to most fully capture the goods of a given community or worldview. Theological context and commitments are central to the formation of such worldviews and a more textured inclusion of such theological considerations is vital for optimal methodological design of religion and health research.

Another concept crucial to more thoughtfully engaging religion and health from a theological perspective is the centrality of community in rightly understanding health. One of the primary distortions propagated by the religion and health movement has been its frequent endorsement of the individualistic excesses of the therapeutic culture, and thus its lack of appreciation of community as a potential agent of health and frequently the most optimal unit of analysis for considering health in relation to religion. Rabbi Weintraub points toward the significance of this lack of appreciation of the centrality of community when he comments in his chapter:

> My teacher and colleague, R. Tsvi Blanchard, in analyzing Maimonides' treatment of the laws of *bikkur cholim* ("visiting the sick"), taught that the essence of reaching out to those who suffer is "shared vulnerability"—the mutual connection of visitor and visitee, not necessarily in having the same troubles, the same diagnoses, or the exact same experiences—but rather a

common link of mortality, of exposure, of need, and of concern, love, and support. The theme of mutual weeping of "healer" and "healee" is the theme of a number of stories about rabbis across the centuries.[8]

This acknowledgment that rabbis across the years have noted the "shared vulnerability" of humanity as the essence that calls the Jewish community to *bikkur cholim* challenges anyone taking the particularity of their Judaism seriously to consider the place of community with thoughtfulness when considering religion and health as a topic of reflection and inquiry.

The intimacy of the Jewish and Christian stories as embodied in this book requires a similar engagement of the role of community by Christians seriously considering religion and health. Wendell Berry would make no claims to be a theologian, but he has noted in his essay "Health Is Membership," in commenting on health, that it is "not just the sense of completeness in ourselves but also is the sense of belonging to others and to our place; it is an unconscious awareness of community, of having in common."[9] He goes on to say, "I believe that the community—in the fullest sense: a place and all its creatures—is the smallest unit of health and that to speak of the health of an isolated individual is a contradiction in terms."[10] While this may seem like a strong statement, in contrast to our commonly received biomedical and cultural worldview that is captive to individualistic interpretations of health, an increased attentiveness to public health paradigms within the inevitabilities of limited resources and a global understanding of health pragmatically calls us to increasingly consider the community as the primary unit of health.

Consonant with Berry's challenges as an essayist and social critic is the Christian theological voice of Norman Wirzba when he says:

> When we learn to accept and bear our pain together, we develop the habits that best equip us to build communities that acknowledge and celebrate our need for each other. When we fully and without rivalry welcome others, even those who seemingly do not have much to offer in return, we recognize our interdependence and learn the arts of sharing, forgiveness, and gratitude.[11]

The outcomes for the measure of health become much richer in possibility when we start to consider the fullness of creation as Wirzba and many others in the theological community would challenge us to include, when assessing health within the frame noted earlier by Kinghorn in his Thomistically derived "science of human flourishing." Along with this richness of outcomes comes the need to more thoughtfully discern how to best measure those components of human flourishing that do not lend themselves to standard quantitative survey methods and analyses that have been typically employed in the religion and health enterprise. If Philip Rieff was correct in his classic critique of the burgeoning therapeutic culture of the twentieth century, *The Triumph of the Therapeutic,* when he states that "ultimately, it is the community that cures,"[12] then a more carefully elucidated understanding of communities formed by religious belief and practices and their particular potential for contributing to health and human flourishing is vital for gaining a better grasp of these relationships.

The religion and health movement has struggled through the years to better understand the associations between religion and health, with a tendency to emphasize the positive relationships more than the negative. Yet it must be acknowledged that both exist experientially, anecdotally, and systemically when we who live within faith communities examine ourselves honestly. While the "mechanisms" for these associations have eluded us to date, enhancing the theological sophistication and engagement within the religion and health work may offer possibilities for addressing this void when appropriated with attention to the issues discussed thus far. Central to the premise of this book is the claim that attentiveness to these issues within the particularity of faith traditions, grounded in communities of faith and practice as represented by Judaism and Christianity, is pivotal if we are going to make real progress in better understanding these relationships. While the field of religion and health is rich with potential if we take the challenges presented by our theological colleagues seriously, concomitant engagement with progress made in science during recent years by colleagues in such fields as genomics and bioinformatics holds promise for even greater advancements. If we can bring enhanced theological considerations regarding religion and health into conversation with these scientific advances without compromising the integrity of either domain, then we will be able to credibly explore possibilities previously only imagined.

POSSIBILITIES

The concerns and possibilities represented within the essays in this book challenge us to consider how we should move forward with systematic inquiry regarding religion and health. While there is much conceptual work and methodological refinement yet to be done, taking seriously the theological concerns expressed here can make a difference. How do we avoid the excessive instrumentalization of religion, sustain the theological particularity of various faith traditions, including the full integrity of their respective views of nondomesticated goods, and develop outcomes of health as related to religion interpreted through the lens of a "science of human flourishing" that is informed by the previously noted theological particularity? This will require an investment of time and resources to date not devoted to this work. Discerning the appropriate domains of particularity of faith and practice by which to develop the methods for the necessary analyses will require collaboration and bridging of disciplines not naturally fostered by our academic guilds and commitments. The potential benefits of such methodological collaboration have been noted before, but the barriers have persisted and have limited us in getting substantively past our cross-sectional, associational studies of religion and health using standard survey data, with all of their inherent limitations. The lack of serious consideration by religion and health researchers of the issues reflected in this book, within the Jewish and Christian traditions, have impeded progress. This void has prevented systematic and substantive comparison of communities of faith and practice so as to better understand how they contribute to health outcomes relevant to the desired goods and sense of human flourishing within their particular traditions.

While it must be acknowledged that delineating the boundaries and defining characteristics of "communities" is challenging and only one of many methodological considerations alluded to within the confines of this essay, the necessity of engaging these issues through a theologically informed lens is critical for future substantive progress within the field of religion and health. Taking seriously the significance of distinctive and faithful worshiping communities and how their particular practices of worshiping together, living together, and caring for one another contribute to health and human flourishing will allow us to gain a much more nuanced and credible capacity to understand and interpret the relationships between religion and health.

Concurrent with the challenge to take the particularity of worshiping and serving communities seriously is the need to take advantage of the potential contributions to be made from recent advances in the natural sciences, particularly genomics, for gaining a better understanding of this relationship. Just as we need to gain a more incisive understanding of the components and potential mechanisms operative in the formation of health within communities of faith and practice through theologically informed inquiry, we need to take advantage of opportunities to better understand the relationship of the particulars of the sociocultural and religious "phenotype" of persons in these communities to the increasingly interpretable genetic information made available through advances in genotyping and bioinformatics processing. The conceptual validation of this synergy between enhanced theological consideration adjunctive to accessing advances in genomics in the service of furthering the religion and health field is consonant with the recent work of the distinguished philosopher Alvin Plantinga, regarding the compatibility of science and religion when he says: "Modern Western empirical science originated and flourished in the bosom of Christian theism and originated nowhere else.... This is no accident: there is deep concord between science and theistic belief."[13]

The possibilities for the religion and health field embedded within recent advances in genomics and bioinformatics, by reversing the notion of genome-wide association studies (GWAS) with a phenome-wide association scan (PheWAS),[14] introduce new horizons that we could only have imagined a few years ago. If we develop a more theologically informed and interpretable sociocultural religious "phenome" with adequate numbers to sort according to particularity of communities of faith and practice and can link this to comprehensive large-scale DNA database repositories for analysis using advanced bioinformatics, then we will be opening a new door of understanding. The religion and health field has the opportunity to make substantive gains in our understandings of gene-environment interactions within the religion and health relationship and potentially contribute to the to-date elusive pathway and "mechanism" question for religion and health. Unquestionable conceptual and methodological challenges loom, but the possible new horizons for the field make it worth the effort.

It seems fitting to end this essay with an offering of hope through the lens of lyrics composed by Debbie Friedman, a leader in contemporary worship within American Judaism of recent decades who died during the last year. Her work was a gift to us all and I have witnessed her ability to draw Jews and Christians together through her music, having been present when she led an auditorium full of Jews and Christians in shared worship with her music:

> *"T'filat Haderech"*
>
> May we be blessed as we go on our way.
> May we be guided by peace.
> May we be blessed with health and joy.
> May this be our blessing. Amen.
>
> May we be sheltered by the wings of peace.
> May we be kept in safety and in love.
> May grace and compassion find their way to every soul.
> May this be our blessing. Amen.[15]

NOTES

1. Quoted from a chapter in the present book: Richard Address, "Contemplating a Theology of Healthy Aging," in *Healing to All Their Flesh: Jewish and Christian Perspectives in Spirituality, Theology, and Health*, eds. Jeff Levin and Keith G. Meador (West Conshohocken, PA: Templeton Press, 2012), 29.
2. Quoted from a chapter in the present book: John Swinton, "From Health to *Shalom*: Why the Religion and Health Debate Needs Jesus," in *Healing to All Their Flesh*, 234.
3. Joel J. Shuman and Keith G. Meador, *Heal Thyself: Spirituality, Medicine, and the Distortion of Christianity* (Oxford, UK: Oxford University Press, 2003).
4. Sigmund Freud, *The Future of an Illusion*, trans. and ed. James Strachey (New York: Norton, 1961), 41.
5. Gerald P. McKenny, *To Relieve the Human Condition: Bioethics, Technology, and the Body* (Albany: SUNY, 1997).
6. Quoted from a chapter in the present book: Stanley Hauerwas, "*Suffering Presence*: Twenty-Five Years Later," in *Healing to All Their Flesh*, 252.
7. Quoted from a chapter in the present book: Warren Kinghorn, "St. Thomas Aquinas and the End(s) of Religion, Spirituality, and Health," in *Healing to All Their Flesh*, 144.
8. Quoted from a chapter in the present book: Simkha Y. Weintraub, "Give Me Your Hand: Exploring Judaism's Approach to the Relationship of Spirit and Health," in *Healing to All Their Flesh*, 106.
9. Wendell Berry, *The Art of the Commonplace: The Agrarian Essays of Wendell Berry*, ed. Norman Wirzba (Washington, DC: Counterpoint, 2002), 144–58, quotation on 144.
10. Ibid., 146.
11. Norman Wirzba, *Living the Sabbath: Discovering the Rhythms of Rest and Delight* (Grand Rapids, MI: Brazos, 2006), 86.
12. Philip Rieff, *The Triumph of the Therapeutic: Uses of Faith after Freud* (Chicago: University of Chicago Press, 1966), 68.
13. Alvin Plantinga, *Where the Conflict Really Lies: Science, Religion, and Naturalism* (Oxford, UK: Oxford University Press, 2011), 266.
14. Joshua C. Denny, Marylyn D. Ritchie, Melissa A. Basford, Jill M. Pulley, Lisa Bastarache, Kristin Brown-Gentry, Deede Wang, Dan R. Masys, Dan M. Roden, and Dana C. Crawford, "PheWAS: Demonstrating the Feasibility of a Phenome-Wide Scan to Discover Gene-Disease Associations," *Bioinformatics* 26 (2010): 1205–10.
15. Debbie Friedman, "*T'filat Haderech*," recorded track included on *And You Shall Be a Blessing* (Sounds Write Productions, 1989).

ABOUT THE CONTRIBUTORS

JEFF LEVIN, PHD, MPH (Editor), is University Professor of Epidemiology and Population Health and director of the Program on Religion and Population Health in the Institute for Studies of Religion at Baylor University. He also serves as adjunct professor of psychiatry and behavioral sciences at Duke University Medical Center.

KEITH G. MEADOR, MD, THM, MPH (Editor), is professor and vice chair of psychiatry, professor of preventive medicine, and director of the Center for Biomedical Ethics and Society at the Vanderbilt University School of Medicine. He also serves as professor in the Graduate Department of Religion.

RABBI SAMUEL E. KARFF, DHL (Foreword), is rabbi emeritus of Congregation Beth Israel, in Houston, a past president of the Central Conference of American Rabbis, and founder of the McGovern Center for Humanities and Ethics at the University of Texas Health Science Center at Houston.

RABBI RICHARD ADDRESS, DMIN, is senior rabbi of Congregation M'kor Shalom in Cherry Hill, New Jersey, and is former director of the Department of Jewish Family Concerns at the Union for Reform Judaism.

RABBI WILLIAM CUTTER, PHD, is Steinberg Emeritus Professor of Human Relations at Hebrew Union College-Jewish Institute of Religion, where he held the Paul and Trudy Steinberg Chair in Human Relations and was professor of modern Hebrew literature and education.

RABBI ELLIOT N. DORFF, PHD, is Sol and Anne Dorff Distinguished Service Professor of Philosophy at American Jewish University, and is AJU's rector. He also serves as visiting professor at UCLA School of Law.

RABBI DAYLE A. FRIEDMAN, MAJCS, MSW, BCC, offers training, consulting, and spiritual guidance through her practice, Growing Older: Wisdom + Spirit Beyond Midlife. She is the author of *Jewish Visions for Aging* (Jewish Lights, 2008).

STANLEY HAUERWAS, PHD, is Gilbert T. Rowe Professor of Theological Ethics at Duke Divinity School and holds a joint appointment at the Duke University School of Law.

WARREN A. KINGHORN, MD, THD, is assistant professor of psychiatry and assistant professor of pastoral and moral theology at Duke University Medical Center and Duke Divinity School.

M. THERESE LYSAUGHT, PHD, is associate professor of theology at Marquette University.

STEPHEN G. POST, PHD, is professor of preventive medicine and director and founder of the Center for Medical Humanities, Compassionate Care, and Bioethics at Stony Brook University. He is president of the Institute for Research on Unlimited Love.

JOHN SWINTON, PHD, is professor in practical theology and pastoral care and holds the chair in Divinity and Religious Studies at the University of Aberdeen.

RABBI SIMKHA Y. WEINTRAUB, LCSW, is rabbinic director of the National Center for Jewish Healing and the New York Jewish Healing Center of the Jewish Board of Family and Children's Services.

INDEX

abortion, 87–88, 253
Abraham, 103, 115
Academic Coalition for Jewish Bioethics, 65–66
Academy of Religion and Mental Health, 7
Acts, 94n35, 207
Adam, 103
Address, Richard F., 260
aegritudo (sickness), 134–35
aging, 52–53, 56–57
AIDS, 20, 21
Akechi, Tatsuo, 126
Akiba, 31–32
Albert the Great, 129
Alcoholics Anonymous
  communitas in, 192–93
  egocentrism in, 194
  God in, 191–94
  healing and, 191–97
  Ontological Generality and, 191–97
  service in, 194–96
  spirituality in, 193–94
  Twelve Steps of, 191–92, 194–96
Alcoholics Anonymous: The Story of How Many Thousands of Men and Women Have Recovered from Alcoholism (Wilson), 192–93, 194
Allport, Gordon W., 7
alone (*l'vado*), 46, 47
Alzheimer's disease, 42–43
American Orthodoxy, 20–21
Amidah, 74
"'And Let Us Make a Name': Reflections on the Future of the Religion and Health Field" (Levin), 186
"And Power Corrupts..." (Lysaught), 184n55
Ando, Michiyo, 126
Angel of Death, 107
anointing, 151–53, 177, 177n5
Another Turn of the Crank (Berry), 244–45
Anselm of Canterbury, 128–29
The Anticipatory Corpse: Medicine, Prayer, and the Care of the Dying (Bishop), 164–65, 249–50
Antoninus, 100
Aquinas, Thomas, 119, 263–64
  Aristotelian method of, 134
  atheists and, 139–40
  on health, 131–37
  on proper and immediate acts, 138–39
  psychology of, 134
  on religion, 137–40, 141–42
  religion and health studies and, 135–36, 140–42
  science, on empirical, 128–31
  on spirituality, 140–42
  theology of, 130–31, 134
  theory of, perceptual, 129–30
  virtues for, 144–45
  virtues of, theory of, 138, 146
Aristotelian method, 134
Aristotle, 132–33
on bodies, 252, 263
texts of, 129
virtues for, 144–45
Asaph, 32
Atchley, Robert, 58
atheists, 139–40
Augustine of Hippo, 128–29, 132, 133
autonomy
  in bioethics, 169–70, 184n59
  Jewish law and, 84–86

autonomy *(cont.)*
rabbis and, 84–85
spirituality and, 185n63
as wild card, 34, 35–36
Averroes. *See* Ibn Roschd
Avicenna. *See* Ibn Sina
avodah (sacred service), 59, 62
ayecha (Where are you?), 26–27, 45–49

b. Abba, Hiyya, 104, 105
baby boom generation, 36–37, 44–49
Bacon, Roger, 250
Bag Bag, Ben, 82
Barth, Karl, 128
Bathsheba, 69
Baum, Gregory, 227
beatitudo (happiness), 132–37
Bellah, Robert, 23
ben bayit (member of household), 110
ben Dosa, Hanina, 109–10
ben Levi, Joshua, 106–7
Ben Sira, 29–30
ben Zakkai, Johanan, 110
Benson, Herbert, 179n11
Berezovsky, Sholom Noach, 63
Berger, Peter, 230, 231, 236
Berry, Wendell, 128, 244–45, 265
Beyond the Relaxation Response (Benson), 179n11
bikkur cholim (visiting the sick), 17, 106, 264–65
Billings, John Shaw, 5
binary, 178n10
spirituality as a mental construct, 156–57
spirituality as formal, 154–56
spirituality as private, 160–61
spirituality as subjective, 157–60
bioethics
autonomy in, 169–70, 184n59
as biopolitics, 184n55
cases in, 180n25
description of, 65
Jewish law applied to, 81–91
leaders and, 70
medical ethics and, 20
religion in, 169–70
spirituality and medicine, similarities to, 169–70
biomedical model, 163
biomedicine, 162
biopolitics
bioethics as, 184n55
biomedicine and, 162
Foucault and, 162, 163, 184n55
governmentality of, 163
spirituality and medicine as, 161–77
biopsychosocialspiritual model
anointing and, 151
biomedical model and, 163
dichotomies and, 154
medicine and, 168, 182n39
psychiatry and, 172–73
religious practices and, 151
Birth Control in Jewish Law: Marital Relations, Contraception, and Abortion as Set Forth in the Classic Texts of Jewish Law (Feldman), 66
The Birth of Biopolitics (Foucault), 184n55
Bishop, Jeffrey, 164–65, 168, 172, 249–52
Blanchard, Tsvi, 106, 264–65
Blanton-Peale Institute, 7
Bleich, J. David, 20–21, 83
bodies, 238n6
Aristotle on, 252, 263
authority of, 248
caring for, 101–2
Christians and, 249, 252
communities, abstracted from, 245
discourses and, 164, 166–67, 182n41
Foucault on, 182n37
humans as, 248
as machine, 154, 244
medicine and, 248–52
shalom and, 236
soul intertwined with, 99–100, 234
soul's relation to, 133, 137
spirit as partner of, 99–101
storied, 244, 250
techniques, 182n40
bodily health. *See* physical health
body politic, 23
Borowitz, Eugene, 84–85

Bradshaw, Anne, 181n32
Brigham, Amariah, 5
b'rit (covenantal relationship), 102–3
b'riut (health), 49
Brooks, David, 192
Brothers, Kyle, 166–67
Buber, Martin, 193, 207

Callahan, Daniel, 66
care of the self. *See* personal health
caregiving, 37–39, 40–44, 62
caritas (charity), 133
Carmody, John, 150, 176–77
Carrette, Jeremy, 124
The Case for Marriage (Waite and Gallagher), 202
Cash, Keith, 156
Cassell, Eric, 249
Cavanaugh, William T., 184n58
Cedars-Sinai Medical Center, 18
Chanukah, 62
charity (*caritas*), 133
chayei-sha-a (the last hours), 40
Chernick, Michael, 42, 43
children, 151
Christian communities, 126–27
Christian difference, 252, 253, 254, 263
Christian theologians, 120–21
Christian theology, 126–28
Christian tradition, 177n5, 178n7
Christianity
  health and, 232
  poor and, 178n7
  religion and health studies and, 123–24, 221–22, 236
  scientific research and, 119–21
Christians
  bodies and, 249, 252
  health and, 232–33, 252–53, 263
  illness, faced with, 150, 254–55
  medicine and, 243, 249, 252, 253, 256
  prayer and, 254
  spiritual well-being and, 126–27
2 Chronicles, 28
Cicero, 138, 139
citizenship (*civitas*), 145
city of God (*civitas Dei*), 133, 145
civitas (citizenship or state), 145
civitas Dei (city of God), 133, 145
clinical trials. *See* research studies
Clinton, Bill, 69
Cohen, Hermann, 72–73
Cohen, Stephen, 85–86
commandment (*mitzvah*), 101–2
communitas (community), 189–90
  in Alcoholics Anonymous, 192–93
  Ontological Generality and, 201, 202, 203–4
communities
  bodies abstracted from, 245
  health and, 244, 264–66
  human flourishing influenced by, 267–68
  medicine and, 244, 246, 254, 255
Communities for All Ages, 61–62
community. *See communitas*
"Compassionate and Comfort Care Decisions at the End of Life" (Union of American Hebrew Congregations), 39
conflict, 210
context
  fundamental ethic and, 41–42
  health and, 124–25
  human actions intelligible in, 147
  of religion and health studies, 4–9
  technology and, 35
  wild cards influencing, 36
1 Corinthians, 238n6, 241n37
Covenant, 86
covenantal relationship (*b'rit*), 102–3
Cruzan, 66

Dameron, Carrie, 165–66
David, 69, 76, 99
Davis, Adele, 20
day of rest (*Shabbat*), 59
deiform, 141
dementia, 42–43
deposit (*eiravon*), 108
depth theology, 89–91
Descartes, Rene, 156
Deuteronomy, 26, 30–31, 40
dignity and sanctity. *See* fundamental ethic

DIP. *See* Distant Intercessory Prayer
discourses, 5–6, 163–69, 182n41, 184n53
Distant Intercessory Prayer (DIP), 203
divine image, 28, 98–99, 101–3, 105
divine love, 197, 210–11
divinity, 23–24
Do the Right and the Good: A Jewish Approach to Social Ethics (Dorff), 67
doctors. *See* physicians
Dorff, Elliot N., 67, 77, 78, 86
dualism
  form v. matter, 154–56
  mind v. body, 156–57, 172
  private v. public, 160–61
  subjective v. objective, 157–60
Durkheim, Emile, 23, 24, 212

Ecclesiastes, 35
Eden, 42
Edwards, Jonathan, 200
eiravon (pledge or deposit), 108
Eisen, Arnold, 85–86
Eisenhower, Dwight D., 70
elderly, 63
Eleazar, 104, 105–6, 109
Ellenson, David, 84–86
Emerson, Ralph Waldo, 207
empiricism, 228–29
end-of-life care, 20–21, 53
  issues in, 66
  Reform Judaism and, 39
  spiritual care in, 127
  transformations in, 181n32
Engel, George, 163–64, 168, 172, 182n39
ethics. *See also* bioethics; fundamental ethic
  Jewish responsibility and, 20
  physicians and, 247–48
  situational, 86
  types of, 65
Ethics of the Fathers (Pirke Avot), 71
euthanasia, 253
Evans, John H., 170
Exodus, 30, 40, 41
expanded science, 237
Ezekiel, 28

FACIT-Sp. *See* Functional Assessment of Chronic Illness Therapy-Spiritual Well-Being scale
faith
  empiricism as, 229
  God and, 22
  healing and, 22
  in Judaism, 111–12
  medicine's relationship with, 151
  science and, 22
  traditions, 209–13, 266–67
faith healing, 177n5
Falchuk, Myron, 250–51
fear (*tira'oo*), 40–41
Feldman, David M., 66
Fifth Commandment, 40–41, 43–44
Finkelstein, Joanne, 184n53
Fishbane, Michael, 83–84
For Love of God and People: A Philosophy of Jewish Law (Dorff), 86
Foucault, Michel, 164
  biopolitics and, 162, 163, 184n55
  on bodies, 182n37
  on governmentality, 163, 181n36
four-humor theory, 130
Fowler, James, 58
Frank, Arthur W., 182n40
Frankl, Viktor, 45
Freedman, Benjamin, 41
Freehof, Solomon B., 40
Freud, Sigmund, 261–62
Friedman, Debbie, 269
Functional Assessment of Chronic Illness Therapy-Spiritual Well-Being scale (FACIT-Sp), 125–26
fundamental ethic, 34–36, 38, 40–42, 43–44
fundamentalism, 212, 213
The Future of an Illusion (Freud), 261–62

Galen, 113
Gallagher, Maggie, 202
Gamliel, 109–10
Gamliel, Rabban, 78, 94n35
Gandhi, Mohandas K., 207
Gawande, Atul, 251, 258n20
gemilut hasadim (giving and receiving care), 62

Genesis, 26–27, 45–48, 97, 115
God, 24, 46, 102–3, 197. *See also* divine image; divine love
actions of, 230–31
as Adonai, 27–28
in Alcoholics Anonymous, 191–94
as Author of *Torah*, 82–84
city of, 133, 145
David and, 99
domestication of, 261–62
existing in horizontal space, 23
faith and, 22
gift of, 234
harmony created by, 99
as healer, 73–74
healing and, 22, 28–30, 32–33, 73–74, 201
humans and, 23, 97–99, 130
as incomprehensible, 147
journey toward, 141
Judaism and, 75
love of, 110, 201, 209–10
as marital partner, 73, 93n16
Meier and, 18, 21–22
moral person created by, 73–74
perspective of, 74–75
physicians and, 31–33
property of, 70
relationship with, 27, 29, 73, 232, 233–34, 260
religion about, 138–39
in religion and health studies, 219
science and, 221
Summa theologiae on, 130
vengeful, 201
vision of, 133–34
will of, 86–87, 90
"God on the Brain" (Groopman), 22
goses (patient close to death), 38–39, 40
governmentality, 163, 181n36
Green, Arthur, 23
Groopman, Jerome, 22, 250–51

Hadas, Moses, 93n27
halakhic formalism, 84–85
Hall, Daniel, 159
Hama, 102–3
Handbook of Religion and Health (Koenig, McCullough, and Larson), 3–4, 238n1
Handbook of Religion and Mental Health (Koenig), 220
Hanina, 104, 108
happiness (*beatitudo*), 132–37
Hartman, David, 20
hashavat aveidot (restoring something lost), 112
Hastings Center, 66
Hauerwas, Stanley, 242–45, 263
Heal Thyself: Spirituality, Medicine, and the Distortion of Christianity (Meador and Shuman), 10–11
on believing, 180n18, 180n21
on modern thought, 182n39
on religion, 180n14
on spirituality, 180n24, 183n52, 185n63
healer, 28
God as, 73–74
healing and, 114
patients and, 114
spirituality and, 114
as surety, 108
wounded, 194–95
healing, 104
Alcoholics Anonymous and, 191–97
changes in, 18–19
definitions of, 24
divine image and, 105
faith and, 22
God and, 22, 28–30, 32–33, 73–74, 201
healer and, 114
Jewish theology and, 23
Judaism's interface with, 15–16, 20–21, 28–34
Maimonides on, 31, 112–13
midrash on, 31–32
Ontological Generality and, 191–97
package, 111–13
potential of "Team," 113
prayer and, 108–10
prayer of, 32
rabbis on, 74
relationship essential to, 105
remedies, 28–29
Torah and, 30, 31, 106–7, 113–14

healing potential of "Team," 113
health, 49. *See also* physical health; population health; religion and health studies
Aquinas on, 131–37
Christianity and, 232
Christians and, 232–33, 252–53, 263
community and, 68–69, 244, 264–66
context and, 124–25
definitions of, 125, 131–32, 224–25f, 232–35, 245–46, 257n10
fetishized, 171
holistic approach to, 27–28
human flourishing and, 124–25, 171, 264
in Jewish community, 70
Judaism's interface with, 15–16, 20, 27–29, 114–15
Maimonides on, 103
medicine influencing perception of, 226
Ontological Generality and, 190–91, 197–207
religion and, 9–10, 136, 190, 197–207, 226, 239n7, 266–68
religion and health studies and, 259, 260–61, 262–63, 264, 266–68
sanctity hazardous to, 178n7
scientific research on religion and, 3–7
as shadow teleology, 132
to *shalom*, 233–34, 260
spiritual, 232
spirituality's impacts on, 114
theories of, 224–25f
Torah and, 70, 74
as virtue, 252
"Health is Membership" (Berry), 244, 265
health technologies, 152–53
heart (*lev*), 46
Heifetz, Milton, 20
Henkin, Nancy, 61
Herz, Marcus, 32
Heschel, Abraham Joshua, 32–33, 46–47
hessed (lovingkindness), 102–3
Hillel, 27, 101–2
Hirsch, Samson Raphael, 102
holiness (*k'dushah*), 49
Holmes, Oliver Wendell, 95n53
Holocaust, 68, 210
honor (*kabed*), 40–41
honor and respect. *See* Fifth Commandment
2 Hosea, 93
hospice. *See* end-of-life care
household member (*ben bayit*), 110
Hugh of St. Victor, 128–29
human(s)
agent, 188–89
as bodies, 248
contexts of actions of, intelligible, 147
divine nature of, 213
God and, 23, 97–99, 130
love and, 214
religion influencing, 214
as restless wanderer, 141
human flourishing. *See also beatitudo*
Christian psychology of, 143–47
communities influencing, 267–68
health and, 124–25, 171, 264
love, as byproduct of, 208
mortality and, 263
in Ontological Generality, 188–89
religion and health studies and, 127–28
science of, 144–46, 263–64, 266, 267
humility theology, 211

Ibn Roschd, 129
Ibn Sina, 129
illness, 106–7, 134–35
Christians faced with, 150, 254–55
Judaism and, 35–36
medicine influencing perception of, 226
Meier and, 18
prayer and, 243
as prison, 105, 116n25
religious archetypes and, 18
stress induced, 205–6
Talmud and, 19
imitating the Divine (*imitatio Dei*), 33, 102–3
imitatio Dei (imitating the Divine), 33, 102–3
institutions, 167
International Center for Health and Society, 203
Internet, 88
investigators, 4–10
Isaac, 103

Isaac (rabbi), 109
Isaiah, 28, 209
Ishmael, 31–32
Israel, 93n16, 107
Israeli Ischemic Heart Disease Study, 202

Jakobovits, Immanuel, 65–66
James, William, 237
Jeremiah, 93
Jesus Christ
  body of, 256
  love and, 188, 189, 208
  religion and health studies and, 219, 235–36, 238n1
  as *shalom*, 235, 240n33
The Jew Within (Eisen and Cohen, S.), 85–86
Jewish authority, asking of (*responsum(a)*), 40, 90
Jewish community, 60–61, 70, 264–65. *See also* Communities for All Ages
Jewish law
  abortion in, 87–88
  application of, wise, 86–91
  autonomy and, 84–86
  bioethical issues, applied to, 81–91
  body of, 86
  change, subject to, 87
  family and community influencing, 68–69
  history influencing, 68
  intellectual property in, 88–89
  Internet and, 88
  Jewish theology influencing, 73–74
  in Judaism, 89–90
  law influencing, 78–81
  leaders and moral models influencing, 69
  legal rulings in, 66–67
  Pharisees and, 94n35
  prayer influencing, 74–75
  precedents in, 87–89
  soul of, 86
  stories influencing, 67–68
  study influencing, 75–78
  values, maxims, theories influencing, 70–73
Jewish Medical Ethics (Jacobovits), 66
Jewish theology, 23, 26–27, 28, 73–74
Jewish tradition, 81–82. *See also* Jewish law
Jewish Values in Health and Medicine (Meier), 19–21, 24
Jews. *See also* Jewish community; Judaism; rabbis
  AIDS and, 20, 21
  baby boom generation and, 36–37
  b'rit of, 102–3
  decisions made by, 84–86
  duty of, 117n35
  as elders, 63
  family and, emphasis on, 68
  Judaism and, 82
  longevity influencing, 26
  Orthodox, 77–78
  spiritual curriculum of, 58–60
  technology influencing, 26
  tradition influencing decisionmaking by, 37–44
  wild cards influencing, 37
Job, 35, 221
Johanan, 104–6, 108
John, 235, 240n33
Johnson, Lyndon Baines, 69
Journal of Religion and Health, 10, 186
Judaeus, Philo, 102
Judah, Rab, 80
Judah (rabbi), 69–70, 107
Judah the Prince, 110–11
Judaism. *See also* Jewish law; Lifespan Judaism; rabbis; Reform Judaism
  faith in, 111–12
  God and, 75
  healing and, 15–16, 20–21, 28–34
  health and, 15–16, 20, 27–29, 114–15
  holidays and festivals in, 59
  illness and, 35–36
  Jewish law in, 89–90
  Jews and, 82
  leaders used by, 69
  longevity and, 26–27
  medical ethics and, 20
  medicine and, 15–16, 27–34
  morality, applied to, 82
  pain and suffering and, 39–40
  practices in, daily, 59–60

Judaism *(cont.)*
  prayer, subjects in, 105–6
  Torah in, 97
  tropes of thinking in, 21
  values central to, 74, 75

kabed (honor), 40–41
Kant, Immanuel, 154
Kaplan, Berton H., 8
k'dushah (holiness), 49
Kegan, Robert, 58
Kennedy, John F., 69
ketubah (marriage contract), 60
Kiddushin, 40–41, 41–42
Kierkegaard, Søren, 187
King, Martin Luther, 200
King, Richard, 124
Kinghorn, Warren, 263–64, 266
2 Kings, 28
Klineberg, Otto, 7
klipot (shards), 54
Koenig, Harold, 3–4, 238n1
  RCOPE and, 165, 183n47
  on religion, 159, 220
the Koretzer, 99
Kraemer, Joel, 112
Krause, Neal M., 203

Lamm, Maurice, 20–21
Langer, Ruth, 44
Larson, David, 173–74
Lash, Nicholas, 124
the last hours (*chayei-sha-a*), 40
law, 78–81
laypeople, 90
learning and teaching (*torah*), 62, 106–7
lev (heart), 46
Levin, Jeff, 170, 186
Levinas, Emanuel, 72–73
Leviticus, 30, 40, 74
Lewinsky, Monica, 69
life, 39
  aging in, 56–57
  eternal, 147
  holistic approach to, 49
  as journey, 201
  love in, 208
  relationships in, 45–46
  science's place in, 143–44
  Torah as, 107
Lifespan Judaism, 57–63
longevity
  baby boom generation expecting, 37
  caregiving influenced by, 37–39, 42–43
  Jews influenced by, 26
  Judaism and, 26–27
  question in, 44–45
  religion influenced by, 49
  religion influencing, 4
  revolution in, 36–45
  society challenged by, 46
  technology influencing, 26
  time given by, 45, 47
  values and, 48–49
love
  aspects of, 213–14
  Christ and, 188, 189, 208
  of God, 110, 201, 209–10
  human flourishing as byproduct of, 208
  humans and, 214
  in life, 208
  in medicine, 244
  in religion, 211–12
  science studying, 214–15
  suffering and, 209
  understanding unlocking, 214
  as unlimited, 211–12
Love Your Neighbor and Yourself: A Jewish Approach to Personal Ethics (Dorff), 67, 77, 78
lovingkindness (*hessed*), 102–3
Luria, Isaac, 54, 55–56, 72–73
Lustig, Andrew, 152
l'vado (alone), 46, 47
Lysaught, M. Therese, 184n55

Maimonides, 20, 32, 72–73
  on caregiving, 43, 44
  on doctors, 112
  on healing, 31, 112–13
  on health, 103
  on morality, 77

patient, on physician and, 33–34
on physicians, 112, 113
on study, 77
Marmot, Michael, 203
marriage, 201–2
martyrs, 208
Maslow, Abraham H., 7, 237
Matthew, 78
McCormick, Richard, 170–71
McCullough, Michael E., 3–4, 238n1
McFadden, Susan, 58
McSherry, Wilfred, 156
Mead, Margaret, 7
Meador, Keith G., 10–11, 128
on believing, 180n18, 180n21
on health, 124–25, 171
on modern thought, 182n39
on religion, 124, 159, 180n14
on religion and health, 179n11
on spirituality, 126–27, 180n24, 183n52, 185n63
"The Meaning of Health" (Tillich), 8
medical ethics. *See* bioethics; ethics
medical technology. *See* technology
medicine, 258n20
as alternative church, 245–46
biopsychosocialspiritual model and, 168, 182n39
bodies and, 248–52
Christians and, 243, 249, 252, 253, 256
communities and, 244, 246, 254, 255
complementary, 20
environment of, 24
faith healing set against, 177n5
faith's relationship with, 151
health influenced by, perception of, 226
holistic approach to, 33
humanistic, 19–20
illness influenced by, perception of, 226
issues in, 21
Judaism's interface with, 15–16, 27–34
love in, 244
religion and health studies influencing, 259
religion's relationship to, 33, 177n3
truth and, 158
"Meeting My Mother Again" (Carmody), 150, 176
Meier, Levi, 15, 24
book of, 19–23
description of, 17–18
illness and, 18
pastoral (care) movement and, 19
question of, 18, 19, 21–22
religious archetypes and, 18
Meir (Rabbi), 109
Menninger, Karl, 7
mental health, 4, 42–43, 75
methodological atheism, 230–31
methodological deism, 230–31
Mi Sheberakh LaHolim (Prayer for Those Who Are Sick), 100–101
midlife, 54–55
midrash (parable from rabbinic tradition), 27, 31–32
Miriam, 28
Mishnah, 71, 83–84, 87, 97–98
Mishnah Nedarim, 31
Mishneh Torah (Maimonides), 43
mitzvah (commandment), 101–2
Moody, Harry, 58
moral person, 67–72, 73–74, 75–81
morality, 77–81
Morita, Tatsuya, 126
mortality, 46, 203, 204–5, 263
Moses, 26, 28, 75, 82
Mount Sinai, 82
Muller, Hermann, 170–71

Naomi, 59
narrative turn, 242, 243
"The Narrative Turn: Thirty Years Later" (Hauerwas), 242
National Institutes of Health, U.S. (NIH), 6, 161–62, 168
neurotheology, 130
New Testament, 78, 94n35, 235
NIH. *See* National Institutes of Health, U.S.
normal science, 6
Numbers, 28

Observations on the Influence of Religion upon the Health and Physical Welfare of Mankind (Brigham), 5
O'Connor, Thomas St. James, 155, 157, 160, 185n70
Okamoto, Takuya, 126
Okon, Tomasz R., 155, 156, 180n20
Ontological Generality
  Alcoholics Anonymous and, 191–97
  altruism encouraged by, 205, 206–7
  benefits of, 189–90
  care of the self and, 197–98
  caveats of, 208–15
  communitas in, 201, 202, 203–4
  divine love and, 197
  healing and, 191–97
  health and, 190–91, 197–207
  hope v. optimism, and, 199–200
  human flourishing in, 188–89
  marriage influenced by, 201–2
  negative behaviors and, 204–5
  prayer in, 203–4
  religion and, 197–207, 209–15
  sin and, 200
  spiritual emotions influenced by, 199–201
  stress, protecting against, 201
Oral *Torah*, 83
organ donation, 39
Orthodox Jews, 77–78
Osler, William, 5

Pagano, Maria E., 195–96
pain and suffering, 39–40, 105, 209
parable from rabbinic tradition (*midrash*), 27, 31–32
Paradise, 106–7
Pargament, Ken, 165, 166, 171, 183n47
Parsons, Talcott, 7
The Pastor (Peterson), 255–56
pastoral (care) movement, 18, 19
patients. *See also goses*
  healers and, 114
  Maimonides on, 33–34
  physicians and, 33–34, 117n31, 246–49, 255
  rabbis as, 19–20
  technology influencing, 251
Paul, 78, 236
peace. *See shalom*
Peck, M. Scott, 58
personal health, 4–5, 197–99
Peterson, Christopher, 145
Peterson, Eugene H., 255–56
Petuchowski, Jakob, 84–85
Pharisees, 76, 78, 93n27, 94n35
physical disability, 4
physical health, 4–5, 101–2, 132, 134–37
physicians
  ethics and, 247–48
  God and, 31–33
  Maimonides on, 33–34, 112, 113
  patients and, 33–34, 117n31, 246–49, 255
  technology influencing, 251
"Physicians and Patient Spirituality: Professional Boundaries, Competency, and Ethics" (Post, Puchalski, and Larson), 173
pikuach nefesh (saving of life), 39
PIP. *See* Proximate Intercessory Prayer
Pirke Avot (Ethics of the Fathers), 71
Platinga, Alvin, 268
Plato, 128–29, 132
Playing God?: Human Genetic Engineering and the Rationalization of Public Bioethical Debate (Evans), 170
pledge (*eiravon*), 108
population health, 4
positive psychology, 144–45
positivism, 227–29
Post, Stephen, 173–74
practices, 59–60, 164–69, 182n42
prayer, 100–101
  Christians and, 254
  of healing, 32
  healing and, 108–10
  for healing into death, 110–11
  illness and, 243
  Jewish law influenced by, 74–75
  Judaism, subjects in, 105–6
  mental health, as important to, 75
  of Moses, 28

in Ontological Generality, 203–4
Talmud discussion of, 109
theurgic, 110
Prayer for Those Who Are Sick (*Mi Sheberakh LaHolim*), 100–101
Prayer of St. Francis, 207
Project MATCH, 195–96
proper and immediate acts, 138–39
prosperity gospel, 261
Proverbs, 207
Proximate Intercessory Prayer (PIP), 203–4
psychiatric disorders, 4
psychology, 134, 143–47
Puchalski, Christina, 185n70
on physicians, 173–74
on spirituality, 154–55, 156, 171, 179n11, 185n63
Pure Unlimited Love: An Eternal Creative Force and Blessing Taught by All Religions (Templeton), 211

quality of life, 4, 39–40
questions
in aging, 53
on divine love, 210–11
existence, fundamental, 26–27, 34, 45–49
in Jewish law, 26–27
in longevity, 44–45
of Meier, 18, 19, 21–22
mortality influencing, 46
in personal health, 198
in religion and health studies, 5, 6–7, 11–12, 187–88, 215, 229–30, 267
for research study, 113–14
spiritual, 35
in spirituality and medicine, 161–62
theological, 26–27
time and, 45

ra'atan (type of illness), 106–7
rabbis, 120. *See also midrash*
on abortion, 87–88
autonomy and, 84–85
fundamental ethic discussed by, 40–41
on healing, 74
Judah the Prince and, 111
laypeople as partners of, 90
legal rulings issued by, 66–67
parable of, 100
as patients, 19–20
on Pharisees, 94n35
religion and health studies approach of, 15–16
on stem cell research, 88
on study, 93n27
teaching of, view of, 76
on *Torah*, 82–84
writings of, 16
Radical Judaism (Arthur), 23
Rahner, Karl, 200
Ramsey, Paul, 170–71
Rashi, 110
ratio (reason), 132–33, 145
Ray, Ruth, 58
RCOPE, 165, 166–67, 183n47
reason (*ratio*), 132–33, 145
The Reconstruction of Humanity (Sorokin), 205
Reform Judaism, 39
Reich, Mordechai, 33–34
"The Relation of Religion and Health" (Tillich), 8
relationships
covenantal, 102–3
with God, 27, 29, 73, 232, 233–34, 260
healing, essential to, 105
in life, 45–46
mortality influencing, 46
physician-patient, 117n31, 251, 253–54
"Relieving Pain of a Dying Patient" (Freehof), 40
religio (religion), 138, 139, 141, 160–61
religion, 180n14. *See also* faith; religion and health studies; religious practices; theology
affections cultivated in, 200
Aquinas on, 137–40, 141–42
in bioethics, 169–70
definition of, 140, 223–24, 231–32
description of, 155–56
emotional self-control taught by, 200–201
empiricism and, 228–29
fundamentalist, 212, 213

religion *(cont.)*
genericization of, 231–32
as global concept, 223–24
God, about, 138–39
as harmful, 212, 213
health and, 9–10, 136, 190, 197–207, 226, 239n7, 266–68
humans influenced by, 214
illness and archetypes of, 18
instrumentality of, 10–11
as invention, 124
longevity influenced by, 4
longevity influencing, 49
medicine's relationship to, 33, 177n3
Meier and archetypes of, 18
as mental construct, 180n21
mental health influenced by, 4
mortality influenced by, 203
Ontological Generality and, 197–207, 209–15
outliers in, 20
personal health influenced by, 4, 198
philosophical positioning of, 153–61
physical disability influenced by, 4
physical health influenced by, 4, 101–2
population health influenced by, 4
proper and immediate acts in, 138–39
psychiatric disorders influenced by, 4
as public, 160–61
quality of life influenced by, 4
religion and health studies and, 219–22, 260–61, 266–68
religious practices and, 153
researchers defining, 123–24
in scientific research, 4–5, 230–31
scientific research on health and, 3–7
secularism influencing, 212
shalom contributed to by, 261
as shopping center, 200
spirituality, distinguished from, 123–24, 141–42, 157, 185n70
spirituality and medicine and, 156, 168–69, 170–71, 181n27
in *Summa theologiae*, 138–39
theology and, 221
truth and, 158–59
ultimate truth and, 220–22
Unlimited Love in, 211–12
virtues used by, 138–39
wars of, 184n58
well-being influenced by, 4
religion, spirituality, and health movement. *See* religion and health studies
religion and health studies. *See also* scientific research; spirituality and medicine; writings
Aquinas and, 135–36, 140–42
changes in, 22–23
Christ and, 219, 235–36, 238n1
Christian theologians on, 120–21
Christian theology and, 127–28
Christianity and, 123–24, 221–22, 236
concepts in, 223–26
conceptual definitions in, 10
context of, 4–9
discourse on, 5–6
explanations and interpretations in, 9–10
as field, 3–4, 5, 6, 7–8, 10–11, 119–21, 125, 187, 215–16
God in, 219
health and, 259, 260–61, 262–63, 264, 266–68
human flourishing and, 127–28
investigators in, 4–10
issues studied in, 6–8
literature on, 153–54, 180n18, 180n21, 219–20, 262–63
mainstreaming of, 20
medicine influenced by, 259
as normal science, 6
pastoral movement in, 18
positivism in, 227–29
possibilities in, 267–69
problems with, 186–87
Proximate Intercessory Prayer in, 203–4
questions in, 5, 6–7, 11–12, 187–88, 215, 229–30, 267
rabbinical approach to, 15–16
religion and, 9–10, 219–22, 231–32, 260–61, 266–68
religious practices and, 152–53
research in, presumptions of, 10–11

researchers in, 146–47, 267
science influencing, 268–69
as science of human flourishing, 144–46
scientific research in, 3–7
symposia examples in, 7
tensions in, 226–32
theology and, 7–8, 229–31, 235–36, 237, 264
virtues in, 144
religious coping, 166–67
religious practice(s)
anointing as, 151–53
biopsychosocialspiritual model and, 151
fetishization of, 171–72
politics of, embodied, 173–77
religion and, 153
religion and health studies and, 152–53
as resistance, 175
spirituality and, 153
spirituality and medicine and, 151
repair (*tikkun*), 54, 56
research. *See* scientific research
research studies
of anointing, 152–53
design of, 4
on heart disease, 202
on mortality rates, 203, 204–5
questions for, 113–14
on sobriety, 195–96
spiritual assessments and, 168
on stress, 205–6
Thomistic principles influencing, 143–47
on volunteering, 206–7
researchers
in religion and health studies, 146–47, 267
religion defined by, 123–24
spirituality and, 123–24, 142
theologians and, divide between, 215
respect (*tirah, tira'oo*), 40–41
responsum(a) (asking of Jewish authority), 40, 90
restoring something lost (*hashavat aveidot*), 112
return to good graces, proper path (*teshuvah*), 75, 81
r'fuah (healing), 49
Rieff, Philip, 266
Robinson, Wheeler, 234
Roe v. Wade, 66
Romer, Anna L., 179n11
ropheh (healer), 28
Rosner, Fred, 20
r'pha (heal), 28
Ruth, 59, 86

sacred service (*avodah*), 59, 62
Salanter, Israel Lipkin, 72–73
sanitas (bodily health), 132, 134–37
sanum (healthy), 134–35
Scherwitz, Larry, 205–6
science. *See also* scientific research
Aquinas on empirical, 128–31
empirical, 143–44
expanded, 237
faith and, 22
God and, 221
of human flourishing, 144–46, 263–64, 266, 267
life, and place in, 143–44
love studied by, 214–15
religion and health studies as normal, 6
religion and health studies influenced by, 268–69
truth and, 158
ultimate truth and, 221
writings in, 5
scientific research. *See also* research studies
Christianity's interface with, 119–21
distorted expectations in, 10–11
empiricism in, 228–29
flaws in, 125
Lifespan Judaism's implications for, 63
physical and personal health in, 4–5
on religion and health, 3–7
religion and health studies, presumptions in, 10–11
religion in, 4–5, 230–31
Seedhouse, David, 224–25f
Seligman, Martin, 145
separation anxiety, 201
Shabbat (day of rest), 59
shalom (peace)
bodies and, 236
Christ as, 235, 240n33

shalom (peace) *(cont.)*
definitions of, 233
health to, from, 233–34, 260
as person, 234
religion contributing to, 261
spirituality contributing to, 261
Shantideva, 207
shards (*klipot*), 54
shattering. *See shever*
Shekhinah (God's Presence), 102–3
Shema, 74
shever (shattering), 54–57
sh'leimut (wholeness), 49
Shogren, Gary, 158
Short Term Life Review, 126
Shulchan Aruch, 30
Shuman, Joel James, 10–11, 128, 243
on believing, 180n18, 180n21
on health, 124–25, 171
on modern thought, 182n39
on religion, 124–25, 180n14
on religion and health, 179n11
on spirituality, 126–27, 180n24, 183n52, 185n63
sickness. *See* illness
Simon the Righteous, 111–12
sin, 200
Sinai Covenant, 73
Slife, Brent, 228, 230
Smith, Dorothy, 181n36
society, 23–24, 46, 80–81
Soloveitchik, Joseph, 117n35
Sorokin, Pitirim, 204–5, 213–14
soul, 99–100, 133, 137, 234
Spector, Stephen, 210
spirit, 99–101
spirituality
in Alcoholics Anonymous, 193–94
Aquinas on, 140–42
assessment of, 164–68
autonomy and, 185n63
baby boom generation and, 36–37
Christian theology and, 126–27
development of, 58–61
emotional self-control taught by, 200–201
fetishization of, 171–72, 185n66
as formal, 154–56
generic, 261–62
healer and, 114
health, and impacts on, 114
health, as measure of, 232
as mental construct, 156–57
mortality influenced by, 203
negative, 171, 185n63
personal health influenced by, 198
physical health and, 136–37
positive, 171, 185n63
as private, 160–61, 180n24
progress in, 24
psychiatry saved by, 172–73
questions in, 35
religion, distinguished from, 123–24, 141–42, 157, 185n70
religious practices and, 153
researchers and, 123–24, 142
shalom contributed to by, 261
as shopping center, 200
in spirituality and medicine, 181n27
as subjective, 157–60
truth and, 158–59
as wild card, 34, 36
spirituality and medicine (field)
anointing and, 151, 177
binaries in, 154–61
bioethics, similarities to, 169–70
as biopolitics, 161–77
challenges in, 175–76
discourse on, 163–64
dualisms in, 154–61
literature on, 153–54, 178n10
questions in, 161–62
religion and, 156, 168–69, 170–71, 181n27
religious practices and, 151
spirituality in, 181n27
theologians edged out of, 175
state (*civitas*), 145
stem cell research, embryonic, 88
story theology, 242
stress, 201, 203, 205–6
study, 58–59, 75–78, 80, 93n27
suffering. *See* pain and suffering

Suffering Presence: Theological Reflections on Medicine, the Mentally Handicapped, and the Church (Hauerwas), 252, 256
description of, 242–43, 245, 246–47
on medicine, 248–49
on physician-patient relationship, 247–48
Summa theologiae (Aquinas), 128
Aristotelian method in, 134
on God, 130
religion in, 138–39
sanitas in, 135
science of human flourishing and, 145–46
Sunday, Billy, 220
Swinton, John, 260
symposia examples, 7

Talmud, 40–41
abortion and, 87
Babylonian, 83–84
ben Dosa in, 109–10
ben Levi in, 106–7
fundamental ethic in, 41–42
illness and, 19
Jerusalem, 83–84
Johanan in, 104–6, 108
prayer, discussion of, 109
on praying for healing into death, 110–11
"Team," healing potential of, 113
technology
context and, 35
Jews influenced by, 26
longevity influenced by, 26
patients influenced by, 251
physicians influenced by, 251
progress in, 24
traditions and, 38–39
as wild card, 34–35
Temple University Center for Intergenerational Learning, 61
Templeton, John, 211
terrorism, 211
teshuvah (return to proper path, good graces), 75, 81
theologians, 128–29, 175, 215
theology. *See also* Christian theology; Jewish theology
of Aquinas, 130–31, 134
caregiving testing, 43
conflict influenced by, 210
depth, 89–91
humility, 211
questions of, 26–27
religion and, 221
religion and health studies and, 7–8, 229–31, 235–36, 237, 264
story, 242
virtues, 145
writings in, 8–9
theory
Aquinas's perceptual, 129–30
four-humor, 130
of health, 224–25f
of virtues, 138, 146
Thomas, Bill, 57
Thomas, Lewis, 22
tikkun (repair), 54, 56
Tillich, Paul, 8, 170–71
time, 45, 47
tirah (respect), 40–41
tira'oo (fear, respect), 40–41
Torah, 40
abortion and, 87–88
God as Author of, 82–84
healing and, 30, 31, 106–7, 113–14
health and, 70, 74
injunctions in, 28
in Judaism, 97
as life, 107
Oral, 83
public nature of, 75–76
rabbis on, 82–84
reading of, 58–59, 100–101
story of, primary, 67
studying of, 58–59, 80
values in, 70–71
Written, 83
torah (learning and teaching), 62, 106–7
traditions. *See also* Christian tradition; Jewish tradition
faith, 209–13, 266–67

traditions *(cont.)*
Jews influenced by, 37–44
legal, 79–80
technology and, 38–39
Treatise on the Religious Affections (Edwards), 200
Trey, Beulah, 57
tribalism, 212–13
The Triumph of the Therapeutic (Rieff), 266
tropes, 21
Tulsidas, 207

ultimate truth, 220–22
Union of American Hebrew Congregations, 39
United Healthcare/Volunteer Match Do Good Live Well Study, 206–7
University of London, 203
Unlimited Love, 211–12

values
Jewish law influenced by, 70–71
Judaism, central to, 74, 75
judgment and, 77
law weighing, 79
longevity and, 48–49
from study, 77
in *Torah*, 70–71
Van Gelder, Paula, 19
Van Ness, Peter, 8–9
Vanderpool, Harold Y., 8, 170–71
Vaux, Kenneth, 8, 170–71
viator (wayfarer), 134
violence, 209–10
virtues
for Aquinas, 144–45
Aquinas's theory of, 138, 146
for Aristotle, 144–45
health as, 252
in positive psychology, 145
in religion and health studies, 144
religion using, 138–39
theological, 145
visio Dei (vision of God), 197
visiting the sick (*bikkur cholim*), 17, 106, 264–65

Waite, Linda J., 202
wars of religion, 184n58
wayfarer (*viator*), 134
The Ways and Power of Love (Sorokin), 204–5, 213–14
Weber, Max, 162
Weil, Andrew, 33
Weintraub, Simkha Y., 264–65
well-being, 4, 126–27, 189
wellness, 55, 101–2
Where are you? (*ayecha*), 26–27, 45–49
White House Conference on Aging, 47
Whitehall Study, 203
WHO. *See* World Health Organization
wholeness (*sh'leimut*), 49
wild cards, 34–36, 37
Wildes, Kevin, 169
Wilkinson, John, 234
Wilson, Bill, 192–93, 194
Wirzba, Norman, 265–66
working definitions, 223
World Health Organization, 131–32, 257n10
wounded healer, 194–95
writings
ancient and medieval, 5–6
empirical, 3
rabbinic, 16
scholarly, 3–4, 5, 6, 151
scientific, 5
theological, 8–9
Written *Torah*, 83
Wurthnow, Robert, 124

Zohar, 72–73
Zoloth-Dorfman, Laurie, 86